AF720137

The Sacred Geometry Materia Medica

Homeopathic Remedies for the New Earth Mind, Body & Soul

Danica Apolline-Matić

First Published in Great Britain in 2026 by Danica Apolline-Matić

978-1-9194555-0-1

Copyright © Danica Apolline-Matić 2021, 2025

danicaapollinematic.com

All rights reserved. No part of this book may be reproduced by any mechanical, photographic or electronic process, or in the form of a phonographic recording; nor may it be stored in a retrieval system, transmitted or otherwise be copied for public or private use, other than for "fair use" as brief quotations embodied in articles and reviews, without prior written permission of the publisher.

The information given in this book should not be treated as a substitute for professional medical advice; always consult a medical practitioner. Any use of information in this book is at the reader's discretion and risk. The author cannot be held responsible for any loss, claim or damage arising out of the use, or misuse of any key of this book or the suggestions made or the failure to take medical advice.

Dedicated to our remarkable solar system, our beautiful planet, our beautiful medicinal plants, trees and all of nature, our beautiful bodies, our remarkable DNA, our incredible electromagnetic field, and my beautiful boy.

For being living proof to me of what I share here.

"There is a rhythm to this Universe that no clock can capture, no calendar can predict, it is the rhythm of the Divine.

It moves not according to your impatience, not by your logic and not by your ego's demands, but by something infinitely wiser, infinitely vaster.
Divine Timing is not late, it is not early and it's never wrong., It arrives like the tide. Not to meet your schedule but to meet your soul's evolution.

When you begin to understand this not as a concept but as a living truth etched into the silence of your being, something inside you relaxes. You stop measuring your life by the ticking of time and start measuring it by the expansion of your awareness."

Dr Wayne Dyer

Contents

Table of Contents

Acknowledgements....13
Indigenous Australian terminology....17
Introduction....19
Phi Mathematics - The Vibration & Mathematics of Love Woven into Sacred Geometry....26
Our Bodies as an Expression of Sacred Geometry & Love....30
Structured Water....32
....33
The Vital Force, Microbiome, and Immunity as Living Sacred Geometry....33
The Fractal Nature of Reality - The Mandelbrot Set....38
Sacred Geometry & The True Nature of Our Vital Force....40
Sacred Geometry & Goethe's Teachings on The Totality of a Person....43
Sacred Geometry as Sarcodes....44
The Masculine & Feminine, Sacred Geometry & the Platonic Solids. 45
Key Themes of the Sacred Geometry Remedies....47
The Constitutional Flower....48
Potencies....52
The Golden Spiral Detox Protocol....56
The Golden Spiral Sarcodes....58
Trademarks & Availability....60
The Golden Spiral....65
The Flower of Life....111
Vesica Piscis....147
The Seed of Life....171
Egg of Life....184
Fruit of Life....198
Tree of Life....214

Grid of Life........ 233
Merkabah........ 249
Torus........ 261
Vector Equilibrium........ 279
The Platonic Solids........ 304
Tetrahedron........ 308
Hexahedron........ 319
Octahedron........ 330
Icosahedron........ 342
Dodecahedron........ 352
Metatron's Cube........ 365
The Bosnian Pyramid of the Sun........ 384
The Pleiades........ 430
Provings & The Fabric of The Universe........ 441
The Trituration Journey........ 443
Epilogue........ 444

Part 1

Background to the Sacred Geometry Remedies

Acknowledgements

There are so many that I wish to express the deepest heartfelt gratitude.

Firstly to some of my greatest teachers - Pythagoras, Paracelsus, Dr Samuel Hahnemann, Dr Melanie Hahnemann, Jerome Whitney, Val Lawrence and Bert Hellinger. Thank you for lighting my way.

To the Anangu, the Indigenous peoples of what the white people know as Central Australia. In particular, thank you to the Watarrka people and all those at Lilla, the lands and ancestors of these beautiful, wise peoples for allowing us to experience and connect with an iota of the magic, wisdom and teachings of the Northern Territory, including at Lilla and Uluru.

Nicki Miller, Meg Humphreys, Natasha Andreo, Shilpa Mehta, Lizzie Martinez, and my dear sister Millie Matić for sharing in the adventure of a lifetime to the Northern Territory during which we triturated most of the sacred geometry remedies in this book, and camped out under the stars in the Outback. We made some of these remedies sitting around a campfire at night, illuminated by the glorious carpet of stars and the Milky Way above us. Waking up with you all under those stars, with Xavier Rudd's *Follow The Sun* as a wake up call on our first morning there will remain imprinted in my heart and soul forever. An extra big thank you to Meg Humphreys who drew on her experiences as a Ranger in the Outback in a previous life to lovingly arrange this magnificent experience for us all. Thank you too to all those at Remote Educational Tours Australia, especially Cara Munn, Reg and Andrew who are tirelessly devoted to honouring and supporting the preservation of the precious wisdoms and cultures of Indigenous peoples across the Northern Territory. My wish is that the Anangu people once again *thrive.*

Ramona Popescu, Rebecca Dove-Thomas, Nicki Miller, Bex White, Rakhee Shah, Michell Childs, Michelle O'Donnell, Natalie Clapham, Rebecca Westbrook, Gail Shaw, Hayley Hurst, Jenie Sparkes, Suzette Knight, Kristina Samoilova, Peter Angel, Mike Andrews, Lisa and Bree for the incredible adventure to the Bosnian Pyramids in March 2025. What a remarkable joyous experience we had, it was beyond my wildest imaginings. Who knew when we set off that we were going to see this remedy connect us so beautifully to the Northern Territory and Uluru.

Dr Semir Osmaganich, a true pioneer in the spirit of Dr Samuel Hahnemann, who has so generously given his time and wonderful encouragement of our work. Dr Osmaganich discovered the Bosnian Pyramids as well as their connection with the Pleiades - indeed has been able to scientifically map out the Golden / Fibonacci Spiral at both, as you shall discover. His quiet dedication to healing the divisions and bringing unification following the years of war in the former Yugoslavia is also truly inspiring to me - and a reflection of the stories told of the Pleiades by the Indigenous peoples of Australia, as I shall share..

All of the students and teachers at the Golden Spiral International School of Homeopathy. Watching each student discover how amazing they are and how powerfully homeopathy heals as we weave together the most beautiful journey of learning, connection, transformation, evolution and expansion is one of the greatest gifts to me in my life. An extra big shout out to the firestarter that is Bex White for lighting the torch of the school that then burst into it's bright and brilliant life. The school and this work exists because of you..

My dear friends who cheerlead me on. Especially Vickie Boyle, Mariana Weigel Munoz, Sophie Joseph, Karen Bell, Wanda Whiting, Amanda Radix, Lucy Setters, Gosia Charysz, Alpa Pabari, Bex White and Krish Surroy. Thank you with my whole heart. I am forever grateful and I love you all.

My beautiful son Reuben. Watching a child grow really is the greatest invitation to see all that sacred geometry represents. Thank you for being there in the beginning, when this remedy journey began, on a cold, blustery Winter Solstice day in 2020 in Greenwich Park, in London, England, when the first remedy in this series - the Golden Spiral - was made. We had no idea where the journey would take us. Thank you for playing your part in the unfolding spiral of my life and for being there at the start of the creation of these remarkable remedies. It's the greatest honour to watch the beautiful unfolding spiral of your life as your Mama.

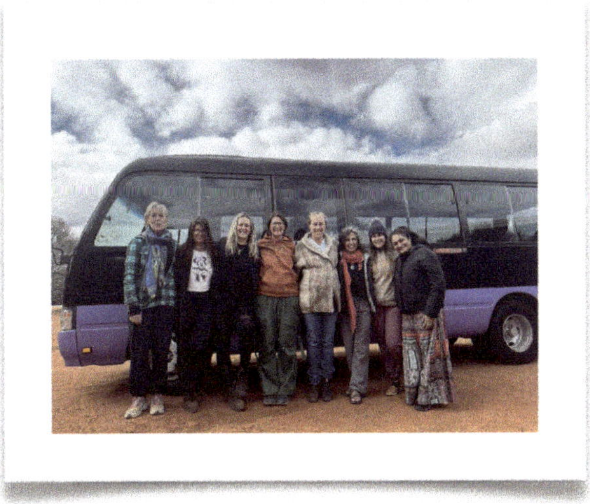

Indigenous Australian terminology

Much of this wonderful journey happened in Australia, in the remarkable Outback. We were extremely privileged to spend time with Indigenous Elders and on Indigenous lands. The term "Aboriginal" is the official term used to refer to Indigenous peoples of Australia. When the prefix "Ab" is placed before a word, it means "not". For example "Abnormal" means "not normal". Aboriginal means "not original".

On our travels, I found myself reflecting on what the effects to the psyche and soul are caused by Indigenous people being repeatedly called "not original"; and having been taught to refer to themselves using this term to; the sense of displacement that such deliberate programming must cause.

Aside from explaining this here, I will not be using the word to describe the Original Peoples of Australia - it is said that, in fact, they are the oldest peoples on Earth. So, I will refer to Indigenous people, and at times the Original people of Australia.

Introduction

As I sit on a beach on the beautiful Balinese island of Nusa Lembongan, watching the sun set majestically with a bright red glow across the horizon, on a day when for the first time in my life I swam with Manta Rays, I am reflecting on the many years these remedies have been in the making.

Many Indigenous peoples around the world tell of the stories of the peoples that first came to the Earth from the stars. We are taught in conventional Western schools that there are two creation stories from which we can choose - the biblical stories of Genesis and Adam and Eve, or Charles Darwin's Theory of Evolution; that we evolved from monkeys.

There is another story that has been written out - that we came from the stars. These are the stories that Indigenous peoples know. We see evidence of this in the world, from the statues in Egypt of the first Ancient Egyptians - the Hathors - whose large elongated skulls and almond shaped eyes make it is easy to see how we may have come from there. The Dogon tribe in Mali in West Africa, another ancient peoples, have their own hieroglyphs - which in fact are symbols expressing the fabric of reality told by their wise elders for aeons; knowledge that we would understand as quantum physics and quantum mechanics. Laird Scranton, a remarkable computer programmer turned hieroglyph detective has decoded the Dogon hieroglyphs and proposes that the Ancient Egyptian hieroglyphs express the same knowledge of the fabric of the Universe; that the hieroglyphs tell of a quantum reality.

We have been taught that we have genetics and genetic ancestors, that our genes are fixed, however brilliant scientific minds like that of Dr Bruce Lipton have been proving that this is indeed not true; that whilst our DNA is fixed, our environment and our thoughts can turn our genes on and off. Dr Zach Bush asks deep questions about how our DNA is formed, and suggests that, in the moment of creation, our DNA is formed in a huge explosion, in the waters of our mother's bodies..

Nobel Laureate Professor Luc Montagnier published research in 2009 showing that highly diluted solutions of water that had contained bacterial DNA still held the memory of the original DNA. He measured how highly diluted water that had contained bacterial DNA emits low frequency electromagnetic signals. These electromagnetic signals could be matched to audible frequencies, which were recorded and then sent from his laboratory in Paris to researchers in Italy. The researchers in Italy played the sound frequencies to distilled water that contained nucleic acids which is what makes up DNA - and the nucleic acids arranged themselves within an hour to form a 98% match to the DNA in Paris - purely from the sound frequencies being emitted. He and his team were then later able to demonstrate the same phenomena with human DNA.[1]

It may be that the moment an egg chooses a sperm, the mitochondria crucial to both to facilitate conception produces water - Source into which DNA from the cosmos can enter.

Sacred geometry is the knowledge of the fabric of reality as expressed by the unfolding patterns created by the mathematics of reality. It comes from the stars, like - I would suggest - we do.

Dr Masuro Emoto was able to demonstrate the expression of sacred geometry through water. He froze water and took photographs of the ice crystals formed as a microscopic level. Water from pure water sources, has perfect geometry - and looks like the beautiful

---

1 Montagnier L, Del Giudice E, Aïssa J, Lavallee C, Motschwiller S, Capolupo A, Polcari A, Romano P, Tedeschi A, Vitiello G. Transduction of DNA information through water and electromagnetic waves. Electromagn Biol Med. 2015;34(2):106-12. doi: 10.3109/15368378.2015.1036072. PMID: 26098521.

snowflakes. That same water, when placed on words like hate, loses it's perfect geometry, and instead indistinct blobs form. Water from polluted sources that doesn't contain perfect geometry, when placed over the word love changes to form the most perfect geometry.

Dr Masuro Emoto and now the brilliant Veda Austin have repeatedly demonstrated the remarkable geometry we can see in water.

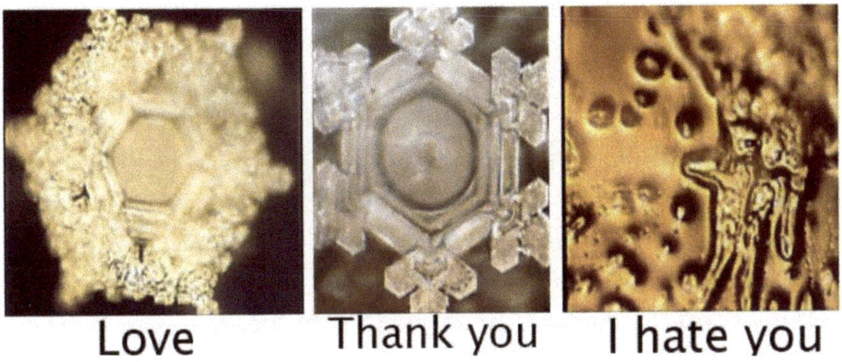

Professor of Biology at McGill University, Gerald Pollack, has been able to demonstrate that there is a fourth phase of water - he calls this Exclusion Zone (EZ) water. It is water that becomes structured in perfect hexagonal lattices - like the honeycombs in which bees make honey. This water isn't H_2O - structured water is H_3O_2. This is the perfect state of water for vitality, wellness and health. H_2O becomes structured H_3O_2 using sunlight, in the mitochondria, which is maintained by the liver, kidneys, heart and the tissues and organs of the body.

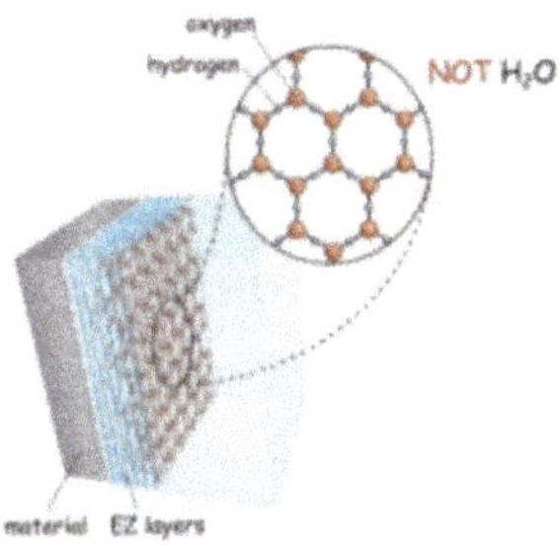

Conventional science now finally recognises that we have a biofield - or, an aura or electromagnetic field, to use other terms that we recognise for this. Our very biofield, when healthy and whole is an expression of sacred geometry. Sacred geometry vibrates with love - as has been measured scientifically by Manfred Clynes, as we shall find out.

To work homeopathically with remedies that are an expression of the patterns of our blueprint - our biofield - is to work with the nature of who we are. It takes us back to our origins from the stars.

Homeopathy is built on the foundations of understanding a person's constitution; who they are at a personality level. What can we achieve when we expand outwards from here and work with who our patients and clients are at a soul level. We are all an expression of energy and the mathematics of life and the Universe. The depth of healing that is possible when we welcome in working at that level - at the resonance of the mathematics and geometry of the cosmos from which we have all come - is remarkable. This is the work of the sacred geometry remedies.

There is another aspect of life that Indigenous peoples understand and respect that is seen in some of the core themes expressed through these remedies.

During my training to become a Family Constellations Facilitator, we were reminded of a fundamental truth by one of my teachers, Francesca Mason Boring. She taught us that Indigenous peoples place *meaning* and *connection* at the centre of life. They understand the perfection of life and the natural world. They know how to approach and deal with challenges by holding space together as a collective. They understand the importance of balance and interconnectedness.

Modern cultures have moved away from meaning and connection being at the centre of life, and instead have placed *materialism* at the centre of life. Much of what we see in the world that is problematic can be understood through this realisation.

Homeopathy fundamentally is a system of medicine that is about restoring balance. This has been historically at a physical, emotional and mental level. We are however evolving and understanding that we have souls, and that we can work at a soul level. The birth of Evolutionary Homeopathy with the help of The Guild has helped us to see this, through their wonderful Meditative Proving remedies. The wonderful work of so many others including Melissa Assilem, Linda Gwillim, Peter Fraser, Kate Birch, Declan Hammond, Dr Michal Yakir, Dr Paul Theriault, Kim Kalina, Sarah Valentini, Reeta Pohjonen, Janey Lavelle and others have continued this evolutionary work.

Evolving the practice of homeopathy to include working at a spiritual, ancestral and on a soul level is I am finding hugely helpful in finding ways to transcend the impact of modern life.

To me, sacred geometry is a true expression of the balance of life and the Universe. As we shall see, sacred geometry is an expression of the mathematics and vibration of love itself. It brings us back to the perfection of life and returns us to the natural order(s) of life.

Sacred geometry can help us to transcend traumas, and I feel have a place in how we work with a wider constitutional picture - for fundamentally, we are an expression of sacred geometry. And so to work with sacred geometry remedies is to work with another aspect of our constitutional make-up, as I will share. Working with sacred geometry reconnects us with our energetic blueprint.

Sacred geometry remedies also return us to the aligned natural order of things, a framework for understanding the world and our place within it - again something that Indigenous peoples understand, and also something that we see beautifully illustrated using Systemic Constellations.

Bert Hellinger the Founder of Family Constellations drew upon wisdoms that Indigenous peoples understand. He taught about what he called the "Orders of Love"; the natural orders in which life expresses itself. All Indigenous peoples understand their versions of their own teachings of the orders of life. Constellations explore what has gone out of the natural order of flow within a system and so there is a disrupted flow, so that the system can be restored to balance once more. For example, Emma might grow up thinking she is the First Child, with all of the energetic and psychological meanings given to a first child. If her Mama, however, had a miscarriage before Emma - this means Emma is not the first child, she is the second. So Emma grows up not in her natural place in the orders of life, and so there can be an interrupted flow in her life. In constellations, we do the work to place people in their natural order so that a natural flow of energy and lie can resume. Constellations also explore where there hasn't been a balance of giving and receiving which also causes a disruption in flow, and also who or what has been excluded from any system - further disputing flow.

Watching constellations in a room, to me, is like watching sacred geometry dance. Constellations reveal truths, invite us to rebalance shadow, restore the natural order of a system and our place within in it so that love and life can flow.

At it's core, this is what sacred geometry is an expression of: a returning to balance, following the natural expression of life and the natural flow of life through us when we are in alignment within our system.

I have seen these remedies bring *phenomenal* changes to people's health, happiness and wellbeing,

My wish is that, as I have seen in the beauty of nature and life today, that these remarkable remedies continue the journey of healing and evolution that we are all on.

August 2025

Phi Mathematics - The Vibration & Mathematics of Love Woven into Sacred Geometry

The following extract explains the mathematics, geometry of this geometric pattern. It is taken from the book *Nature's Medicine Code.*[2]

All sacred geometry contains Phi mathematics. What is Phi?

"Phi, symbolised by the Greek letter ϕ, has a value of 1.61803399 known as the Golden Number, Golden Ratio or Golden Mean (or 1.618 for short). It is Pythgoras (570-495 BC) was an Ancient Greek teacher who invented mathematics and arithmetic – the basics of mathematics that we still learn today. He practised in the days where there was no separation between mathematics, science, music, philosophy and astronomy, and he studied and taught all of these. These subjects were understood to be linked to each other during his life 2,500 years ago, and a greater understanding is emerging that he and others who taught in this way were onto something.

Pythagoras studied the vibration of strings as he plucked them on a musical instrument called a lyre. In those days, 7 was considered to be the "magic number" for everything. Music was played using only a 7 tone scale. It was a mark of how respected Pythagoras as a teacher was, that he was successfully able to introduce another number of significance that altered the cultural perceptions of his time.

He identified that, when playing a 7 note scale, it is possible to

2 *Nature's Medicine Code* (2nd Edition) by Danica Apolline-Matić (2024)

create a perfect harmony by adding an extra tone - a small half-step after the 4th note. Even though he was going against the accepted wisdom of the ancient Greeks – that the number 7 is sacred – adding this extra note makes an octave. The perfect octave creates what Pythagoras defined as *harmonia.*

The addition of this "fifth", as this special note is called, leads not only to harmony, but also brings with it a mathematical ratio. Octaves and harmonies have embedded within them a remarkable number: the Golden Number Phi - 1.618.

Manfred Clynes was a concert pianist who embraced a scientific career so that he could find out about the connection between music and emotion.

Manfred found that, irrespective of cultural, religious or racial differences, we all create emotions in the same ways. Emotions, it turns out, are emitted in waves. It turns out that the wave patterns of love are related to Phi – to 1.618. Anger and hate send out different wave patterns that do not contain Phi. Waves of love encourage life to grow and unfold, like the unfurling petals of a flower or the unfurling of our limbs in the womb. Waves of hate, on the other hand, do not contain the magic number of 1.618 and destroy. He published his work in his book *Sentics: The Touch of Emotions.*[3]

The Fibonacci Sequence

Another mathematician - a genius called Fibonacci - lived around 1000 years ago, during the "Middle Ages" in the Italian town of Pisa. Fibonacci discovered a mathematical sequence of numbers that when drawn into a pattern forms the Golden Spiral, or Fibonacci Spiral, which contains the number Phi.

3 https://www.kirkusreviews.com/book-reviews/a/manfred-clynes/sentics-the-touch-of-emotions/

The Fibonacci Sequence goes like this:

Start at 0 and count up, each new number is the sum of the previous 2 numbers. So
the sequence goes like this:
0+1 = 1
1+1 = 2
1+2 = 3
2+3 = 5
3+5 = 8
8+5 = 13
8+13 = 21

and so on, so the sequence looks like this:
0,1,1,2,3,5,8,13,21,34,55,89,144, 233......

If you divide one number in the Fibonacci sequence by the number before it, then you get Phi at any point from 89 onwards– or at the smaller numbers, a number very very very close to Phi. The further along the sequence you go, the closer and closer to the exact number of Phi you come......"

The Golden Spiral, is a beautiful example of how we can see the Fibonacci sequence visually. The numbers in the Fibonacci sequence are drawn onto graph paper, with each number representing the size of the square a line is drawn in – so starting at 0, then drawing across 1 square, then 1 square, then 2 squares, then 3, then 5, then 8 and so on carrying on using the Fibonacci sequence numbers, they form a pattern – it is a perfect ever growing spiral.

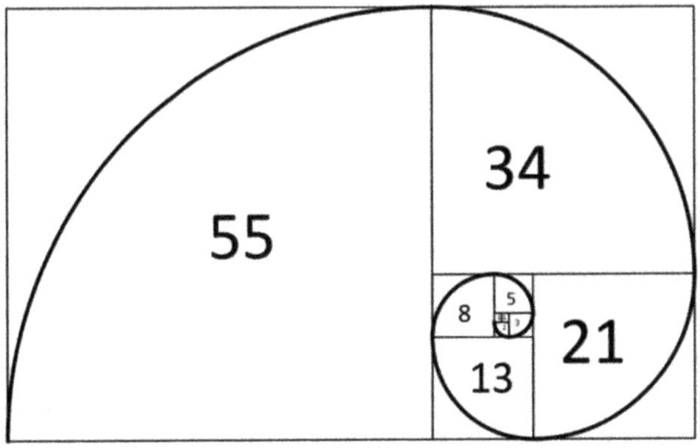

The Golden Spiral emerges out of the Flower of Life.

The Flower of Life is a sacred geometry symbol made from "19 intersecting circles spaced evenly from each other that reveal an intricate pattern of overlapping symmetrical flowers". This is the 2D representation of the Flower of Life, and of course we are 3D beings. However the Flower of Life gives us the blueprint from which all of the other sacred geometry, Metatron's Cube and all the Platonic solids emerge, as you will read in the Flower of Life proving.

I would suggest that the Flower of Life is the Mother - the Divine Mother - from which all life emerges.

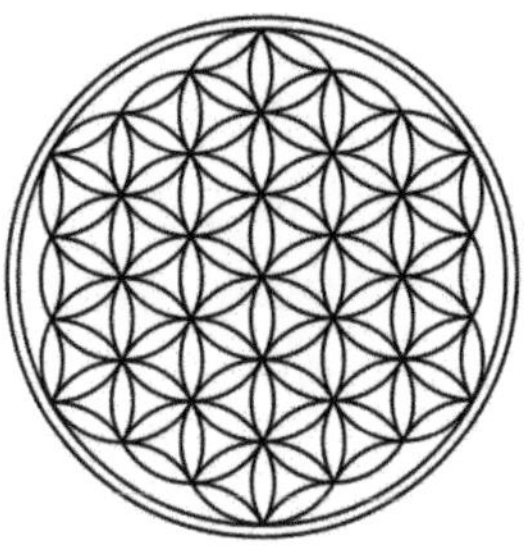

Our Bodies as an Expression of Sacred Geometry & Love

Everything in nature is an expression of sacred geometry. A beautiful example of this can be seen when looking at the Golden Spiral in nature. There is a longer list of examples in the write up of the Golden Spiral, however just to give an idea, we can see the Golden Spiral:

| The arrangement of faces, in particular the positioning of our mouth and nose
along with our eyes and chin
| The proportions of the uterus
| In the spirals of the DNA
| In the growth and unfolding of leaves
| How blood flows through blood vessels
| How hurricanes and tornados travel
| How currents flow in seas and oceans
| In the formation of ice crystals and snowflakes
| How planets in our solar system orbit each other as they travel through the
galaxy
| In how electrons flow around the nucleus of an atom[4]

- How the energy of balanced, healthy chakras flow
- How the soul enters and leaves the body

In fact, researchers at MIT in 2020 were able to observe what happens at the exact moment when an egg is fertilised. They found that biochemical waves travel across the egg - in particular spirals rippling out as the egg grows. The image presented with the research is remarkable. The video of what

---

4 Winter, D, Donavan, B., and Jones, M. (2012) Compressions, The Hydrogen Atom and Phase Conjugation

they saw is remarkable, and be watched using links below. Spirals emerge into the toroidal field.[5]

As we shall come to understand, it isn't just the Golden Spiral that we see expressed in the body, but all sacred geometry can be seen in our bodies.

5 Tzer Han Tan, Jinghui Liu, Pearson W. Miller, Melis Tekant, Jörn Dunkel & Nikta Fakhri Topological turbulence in the membrane of a living cell. March, 2020 https://doi.org/10.1038/s41567-020-0841-9

Structured Water

I have already touched upon the remarkable work of Professor of Biology at McGill University, Gerald Pollack.

Professor Pollack has been able to demonstrate that there is a fourth phase of water - he calls this Exclusion Zone (EZ) water. It is water that becomes structured in perfect hexagonal lattices - like the honeycombs in which bees make honey. This water isn't H_2O - structured water is H_3O_2. This is the perfect state of water for vitality, wellness and health. H_2O becomes structured H_3O_2 using sunlight, in the mitochondria, which is maintained by the liver, kidneys, heart and the tissues and organs of the body.

This is geometric water; water that is arranged in a way that reflects the mathematics of life and the Universe.

Given that we are 70-80% water, ensuring that the water we have access to is energetically aligned with the vibrations of the cosmos and life itself becomes crucial to maintain health and vitality.

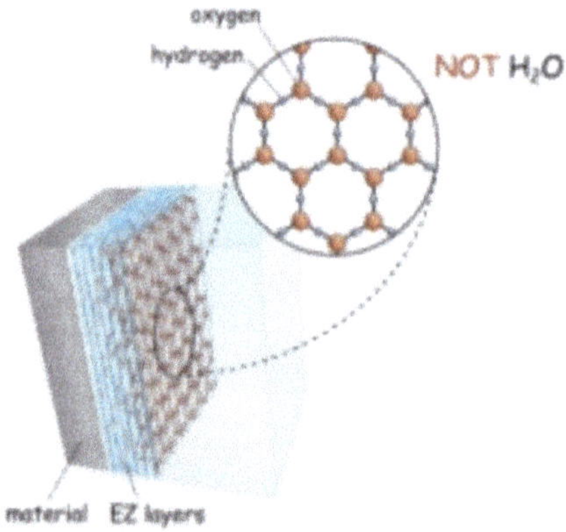

The Vital Force, Microbiome, and Immunity as Living Sacred Geometry

One of my greatest joys in teaching at the Golden Spiral International School of Homeopathy® has been journeying deeply with Anatomy & Physiology in a new way; through a lens that includes sacred geometry, quantum biology & metaphysics too.

My greatest eureka moments have come from teaching the cell, mitochondria, circulatory, digestive, hepatobiliary and immune systems.

As I have felt into the systems that weave us into existence, I have been able to understand some of the patterns and geometric structures that are an expression of this in a whole new way.

Before I share what I have come to understand about the Vital Force, I am going to share what I have come to understand about the nature of the Digestive and Immune Systems.

We are an ecosystem, not an individual

Our bodies - and our energy fields - are in the shape of a ring donut - one with a hole in the middle. The "hole in the middle" of our physical bodies is the digestive tract that runs through the centre of our bodies from our mouth to our anus. In the same way that we put moisturisers on our skin and the ingredients are absorbed into our bodies, the same thing happens with ingredients from food being absorbed into our bodies through our digestive tract.

Covering the surface of our skin, and lining the digestive tract is an ecosystem akin to a forest; made up of bacteria, fungi, viruses, protozoa, parasites - a trillion-member community co-creating health. Like a woodland's mycelial web, the microbiome is a distributed communication network. It trades nutrients, shapes immunity, and sends biochemical "messages" that influence mood, appetite, and perception.

Life speaks in spirals - from how the soul enters and leaves the body to chakras to the DNA to the mitochondria to spirochaetes. Spirochaetes are corkscrew shaped bacteria that we meet in the mouth. They are important in detoxification (the spiral detoxifies; spirals out what we don't need), however they have been demonised as the cause of tooth decay.

Like with the entire ecosystem, they can grow out of control and out of balance with the ecosystem when their environment isn't held in harmonious symphony - for example when the pH of the mouth becomes too acidic, which easily happens when too much sugar is consumed.

Along come antibacterial mouthwashes, and hand sanitisers, antibiotics, chlorinated water which all destroy the spirochetes and the other species of bacteria that are part of our ecosystem, and so we can no longer effectively detoxify.

The estimates of how many species of bacteria we have in the human varies widely from 500-1000 species, all the way up to 10,000. Whatever the number, it is a delicate balance.

What there seems to be is agreement that human cells are not just what makes up being human; that there are at least as many bacterial cells. Add to that fungal cells and viruses, not to mention protozoa and parasites, and it is understandable how Thomas D.

Luckey in 1972 proposed that our human cell count may be outnumbered by 100 to 1 at least by our microbiome[6], however more recent estimates still suggest a 1:1 ratio. When we consider that we have an estimated 39 trillion cells, that's still a pretty impressive amount of fungal cells and viruses, not to mention protozoa and parasites making up our microbiome,[7,8]

So we are an ecosystem, not an individual!

Consciousness is not a property of individuals, but a field of relationship, and we see that absolutely in the work of constellations. Microbes and mycelia are not separate beings but important components of a collective being.

Are we actually in service to nature?

Now comes the question, are we actually in service to nature rather than nature being in service to us? We tend to think of ourselves living on the earth with the earth being in service to us.

There is a school of thought proposed by some biologists and thinkers called *distributed intelligence*. According to this school of thought, together with our microbes, we form a single ecological unit. Our sense of self includes not just human cells or consciousness, but cells and consciousness of our entire microbial community.[9]

---

6 Luckey TD. Introduction to intestinal microecology. Am J Clin Nutr. 1972 Dec;25(12):1292-4. doi: 10.1093/ajcn/25.12.1292. PMID: 4639749.

7 Ron Sender, Shai Fuchs, Ron Milo,
Are We Really Vastly Outnumbered? Revisiting the Ratio of Bacterial to Host Cells in Humans, Cell, Volume 164, Issue 3, 2016, Pages 337-340,

8 Ron Sender, Shai Fuchs, Ron Milo: Revised estimates for the number of human and bacteria cells in the body, bioRxiv 036103; doi: https://doi.org/10.1101/036103

9 https://medium.com/predict/who-exactly-am-i-05f6369133e2

Are the decisions we make really *our* decisions as people? Are our ideas our own? Or are they an expression of the collective voice of our ecosystem?

I invite you to hold in wonder the possibility that we are a donut of an ecosystem, a microbiome that includes bacteria, fungi, viruses, protozoa and parasites living in balance with each other, expressing themselves through vibration, through sacred geometry, through colour, through sound, through Phi (1.618) - the vibration of love - and that we are in service to all of this as part of being in service to Mama Gaia, our skin and digestive tract being the interface through which all of this communication is received.

And that our Vital Force is an expression of the collective vibration of all of these as one. And all of these are an expression of the Mandelbrot Set that we've been learning about - the equation that results from where chaos and order meet, and the Golden Spiral - the spiral of life - emerges. In other words, one giant fractal of life, unfurling and expressing itself through the unfolding spiral of life, and the mathematics of love.

Our gut feeling as the collective voice of our ecosystem

Our gut feeling - that inner knowing - that propels us forward one way, or stops us going in another.......what if that is the one collective voice of our microbiome; our ecosystem - the symphony that plays and includes the conductor (the immune system) guiding it.

Bringing balance to "The Force"

I love a *Star Wars* analogy; I love *Star Wars*. I think it teaches us so much about life. I love that it taught us that there is "The Force", as Obi Wan explained to Luke Skywalker: "The Force is what gives a Jedi his power. It's an energy field created by all living things. It surrounds us and penetrates us. It bings the galaxy together."

The Force is "an energy field created by all living things". Together.

The Force is created by the forest, or orchestra of our microbiome. Antimicrobial products literally destroy the forest; affecting the crucial mycelial web as well as the other plants and trees that make it up. It can and does grow back quickly when given the space to do so.

What shapes do they form?

From the spirals of the spirochaetes, the spirals in our mitochondria, the spirals in our DNA and in the DNA of bacteria, we are a symphony of spirals, and also other geometry - the torus, the toroidal field, vector equilibrium, the flower of life, the dodecahedron and more.

The Fractal Nature of Reality - The Mandelbrot Set

The Mandelbrot Set is a fractal that emerges out of a mathematical equation.

The equation comes out of Chaos Theory and measures the point at which order and chaos meet.

That mathematical equation has been typed into computers and a visual pattern created. The image that results from the Mandelbrot set shows how, in everything, there is a repeating expression of the same pattern. When you zoom in to one part of the picture, you find the whole pattern is repeated again within it. No matter how much you zoom in, you see the same pattern within the original pattern you looked at.

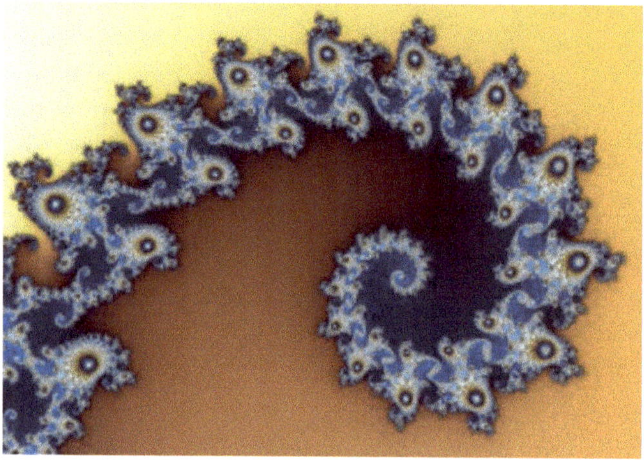

Where order and chaos meet, the Golden Spiral emerges. Too much order, and the Golden Spiral cannot emerge, too much chaos, and also the Golden Spiral cannot emerge.

Indigenous tribespeople all learn to live with the wisdom and balance of order and chaos. In the Western World, we live with an attempt to over-order everything - this suppresses us, and so the Golden Spiral cannot emerge. This is the Empire in *Star Wars* - "We must have ORDER!". It literally squeezes the life out of everything.

There are wonderful places in the world where there is less suppression, and so much more that is *alive* - places that are full of potential expressing themselves; places where some chaos can found, which means magic can erupt into being. Glastonbury Festival is one of those places to me. The Mandelbrot Set in action.

Sacred Geometry & The True Nature of Our Vital Force

"(...)The totality of these symptoms is the *outwardly reflected image of the inner wesen* [essence] *of the disease, that is, of the suffering of the life force*(...)." §7

"In the healthy human state, the spirit-like life force (autocracy) that enlivens the material organism as dynamis, governs without restriction and keeps all parts of the organism in admirable, harmonious, vital operation, as regards both feelings and functions, so that our indwelling, rational spirit can freely avail itself of this living, healthy instrument for the higher purposes of our existence." §9

The Organon (6th Edition)

The Vital Force is an invisible field of energy that organises life into harmonious patterns - it is the geometry and expression of love. I would suggest that the Vital Force is a dynamic energy that moves in spirals - as the unfolding Golden Spiral - as we see at the very point of conception, as discovered by the MIT scientists in 2020.[10]

It moves us forward in life. I would suggest that the Vital Force IS the sacred geometry of the Golden Spiral moving us through life; the unfolding fractal spiral. It may flow and form into the Toroidal field - the Torus, which is our energy field, which in turn when whole expresses the geometry of the Flower of Life.

---

10 Tzer Han Tan, Jinghui Liu, Pearson W. Miller, Melis Tekant, Jörn Dunkel & Nikta Fakhri Topological turbulence in the membrane of a living cell. March, 2020 https://doi.org/10.1038/s41567-020-0841-9

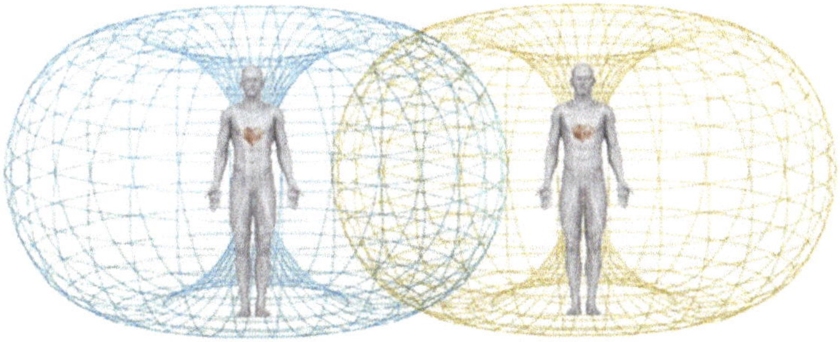

I would suggest that the true nature of the Vital Force as it flows through life is expressed as a collective Golden Spiral, a weaving of all of the spirals found in our ecosystem, just like the fractal that the expression of all of life. It may then flow into a collective Toroidal Field (Torus) made of our entire ecosystem, but that at its core, it is always an expression of the Golden Spiral and the Flower of Life.

If we could "see" the Vital Force, I would suggest that this is what we would see. The Golden Spiral fractal when the magic of what happens when both order and chaos, when lines and curves or the masculine and feminine meet. When we are healthy, the spiral expands with a beautiful emerging flow, in rhythm with nature. When we fall ill, it loses its coherence and geometry, as does our toroidal field.

Healing is the restoration of our natural sacred geometry; the Golden Spiral, our Toroidal Field expressing the Flower of Life, coming back into alignment as a whole.

Sacred Geometry & Goethe's Teachings on The Totality of a Person

Dr Hahnemann was influenced by the work of the famous German polymath Johann Wolfgang von Goethe (1749-1832). Dr Hahnemann wasn't the only leader influenced by Goethe's teachings; the great anthroposophical leader Rudolph Steiner, philosopher Georg Wilhelm Friedrich Hegel and Carl Jung, known as the "father of modern psychology" also were.

Goethe described how there are 4 aspects to a whole person:

- The body *Körper*
- The mind *Gemut*
- The soul *Seele* (this is where we just are who we are; our place of being)
- The spirit *Geist* (this is our connection to Source / some higher spiritual aspect). In essence this is our connection to God (or Source, or Divinity, whatever you might call the wonderful unconditional love from which we are all said to have come), or to use Sigmund Freud's psychoanalytic definition, the *superconscious*.

Dr Hahnemann described how diseases were caused by the "spiritual dynamic mistunement of the organism's life", and how, the material organism and dynamis are a unity, but that thought separates them to facilitate comprehension.

Dis-ease, therefore, is caused by the disquiet that happens when the Mind (*Gemut*) does something that isn't aligned with the Spirit (*Geist* or God, or the Superconscious); where there is a gap between the Mind and the Spirit.

In other words, our highest aspect knows what is wonderful for us and what isn't; what enables us to thrive and flourish and helps others and the world around us thrive and flourish - and what doesn't. It knows when we do wonderful things for others, and when we don't. And when we don't, even when our mind tries to justify it, some inner subconscious part of us knows and *feels* uncomfortable, and feels out of integrity. That disquiet; that *dissonance* as psychologists would describe it, creates the perfect conditions for dis-ease to set in.

Our Spirit *knows* when we act in ways that are not in alignment, so when we don't, that forms a *gap* between the Mind and the Spirit, and that GAP creates a dissonance, a discomfort where disease can set in.

The Sacred Geometry remedies have at their core *alignment*. They invite a weaving of the different aspects that make up the totality of a person - in Goethe's terms, the *Körper* (body), *Gemut,* (mind), *Seele* (soul) and *Geist* (spirit). Where is disconnection, they bring connection. All of the sacred geometry remedies do this in their own ways, but I especially look to Golden Spiral, Flower of Life, Torus, Vector Equilibrium, Dodecahedron and Metatron's Cube. In fact, I would suggest that when complete and whole, the Totality of a Person is most completely expressed by the Flower of Life.

Sacred Geometry as Sarcodes

I feel that the Golden Spiral is the geometric sarcode of the DNA and the Flower of Life is the geometric sarcode of the cell, and of the energy field. This is how I work with them, and prescribe them.

The Masculine & Feminine, Sacred Geometry & the Platonic Solids

"The straight lines and angles of geometry symbolise the limitations of our physical world, while the curves and circles symbolise the infinite possibilities of the spiritual realm." — Hasidic teaching

The Platonic Solids are Sacred Geometry, however I am presenting them in two sections separately. Why?

The Platonic Solids were originally discovered by Pythagoras (c 580 BC - 500 BC) an Ancient Greek polymath and philosopher but it was Plato (427 BC - 347 BC) another Ancient Greek philosopher who really brought them to our awareness.

The purpose of the masculine is to hold space for the feminine to move, to flow, to whirl, dance, create, express. It is the role of the masculine to see the beauty in the feminine - something I first heard Dr Zach Bush describe, at the same event where Telfer Montgomery showed us how the masculine is straight lines, and the feminine is swirls and curves. I have reflected on this a lot, and am in awe of how we see this expressed in our bodies; the straight lines of the body of most men and the curves of the bodies of most women.

This is a wonder to behold. How does it look in relation to sacred geometry?

The Platonic solids create the structure of the Universe. They are made of a series of straight lines that form polygon shapes (with equal lengths of each side) that are then joined together to form shapes that define the structure of reality. This is the masculine holding the outer edges, the perimeters that form the boundaries of space and time.

They are all, however, birthed out of the Flower of Life; the egg - which needs the sperm to meet before the Golden Spiral emerges in the moment of conception. The Flower of Life is a feminine concept - like the Mother of all geometry birthing life before her.

The sacred geometry that I describe in the Sacred Geometry section are the feminine expression of flow, dancing, expressing life in the most beautiful ways within the boundaries of the Universe. These include the Golden Spiral, the Flower of Life, the Egg of Life, the Seed of Life, the Tree of Life and more as you will discover.

Between them, we see a beautiful order in the expression of life: the masculine structured lines of the Platonic solids holding the boundaries of space, time and reality whilst the feminine sacred geometry dances within, her beauty expressing life witnessed by the masculine.

All of them born out of the Flower of Life; the Divine Mother.

I find it a truly beautiful reflection of the unfolding fractal of life where we see lines for the masculine and curves for the feminine, starting with the nature of the Universe, coming right down to the miracle of our bodies.

Key Themes of the Sacred Geometry Remedies

The following key themes apply to the whole series of Sacred Geometry Remedies, including the Platonic solids:

Alignment
Harmony
Balance
Empowerment
Sovereignty
Integrity
Truth
Wisdom
Life Purpose / Soul's Purpose
Healing
Transforming personal
Healing ancestral trauma
Transcending the patriarchy
Transitions - Birth & Death
New Earth
New Human
Peace
Love
Connection
Source

The Constitutional Flower

I have developed a model that I hope brings a wonderful perspective on how we understand our constitution. I have called this the Constitutional Flower.

Many of us understand that originally we were thought of as being only being one constitutional remedy. We all still at times meet people who clearly have one standout constitution, such as Arsenicum or Calc carb or Pulsatilla. We have evolved through time and become much more complex in some ways - perhaps in response to the complexities of modern life, or maybe because we ourselves are evolving. It may be due to a multitude of reasons, however what is clear is that some of us can be an amalgamation.

I love seeing it as a Venn diagram of 2, 3, 4 remedies - this approach was first introduced to me by Lynne Russell.

I have sat with this for the years since, and I am going to share a model I hope you find beautiful.

I've got a feeling that we've got at our foundation a constitution that's made of a combination of each of the plant, animal and mineral kingdoms. When I look at my patients, I can't think of any time I've ever seen someone who is definitely a blend of constitutional remedies who will be a combination of two or three plants, or two or three minerals, or two or three animals. What I do see is often everyone has a plant aspect, a mineral aspect, and an animal aspect. We have elements of all of the kingdoms within us - even if one predominates over the others.

We all need love and nurture that we see in the plants, we all have a need for structure and order that we see in the minerals, and we all need some kind of social structure, relationships, sexual expression, and to protect or be protected as we see in the animal kingdom.

Now I'm going to go a little deeper here and make a suggestion for something else. What happens if we consider that we're not just made of a plant, an animal, and a mineral? What happens if we consider that we might also be made of an imponderables? If you like, the more spiritual remedies, the meditative provings, for example, the remedies that speak to the soul. I don't include the sacred geometry remedies here, I will explain why shortly - they DO have a place, but not in the Venn diagram of petals that make up the constitutional flower.

In the following diagram, I am going to suggest the following:

- Each of the four petals represents one of the following: animal remedy, plant remedy, mineral remedy and imponderable remedy - this makes up the person's constitution.
- Then around the constitutional flower can be listed the remedy states someone can go in to that are relevant to that kingdom. Eg Calc carb going into a Pulsatilla state
- Each flower has a stem through which it emerges, and at the end of its life once the petals have fallen away, it is the stem that remains that returns to the Earth. I would suggest that, for most if not all of us, our stem is Calc carb. We emerge into life through Calc carb - a time when home, stability, and being slow and steady, calcium to help us grow is a fundamental for our growth. Eventually, at the end of our lives, if we live long lives, we return to a Calc carb state,

What about sacred geometry?

We all have Golden Spiral and the Flower of Life and all of the geometry at our core. We have our constitutional remedies that speak to our *personalities,* and then we have the sacred geometry remedies which are like the constitutional remedies that speak to our *soul.* We are all made of the sacred geometry remedies, and so, at our core - at our *soul* level, our blueprint or Being, the sacred geometry remedies speak to us all.

So taking sacred geometry remedies is like working constitutionally at a *soul* level. Sacred geometry remedies speak to everyone's soul level constitution - this is the energy blueprint that all of us has at our core.

So what does this look like?

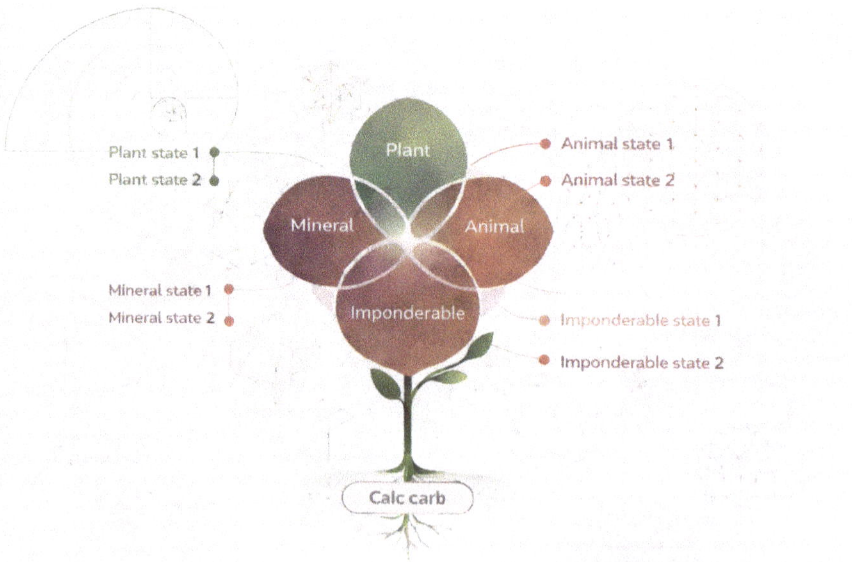

An example here could be someone whose constitutional plant remedy is Lycopodium, but they can go into a Staphysagria or a Thuja state, depending on the situation.

I see each prescription itself as a work of art. I imagine the different frequencies of vibration of each remedy that goes into the prescription. I get a sense intuitively of whether they fit together like a beautiful painting or a beautiful piece of music.

So if you were to draw your constitutional flower, what would yours look like?

Potencies

This work is born of love - a love of and dedication to the brilliance of mathematics, and to the exquisite nature of the Universe and to life itself. I hope you can already feel my profound awe and wonder with which I share some of the magic of the Universe.

I am usually a high-potency bunny. When taking all other remedies, my favourite potency for myself is a 50M. When working with patients who are moving through great trauma (one of the areas of great interest to me), if their vital force can take it, I will give 1Ms, 10Ms and 50Ms - especially for the big karma and life and soul clearing remedies including the *Meditative Proving* remedies. The Golden Spiral Sarcode Series that I have made contain sarcodes at a 1M because I have found 1M to be a wonderful potency for regulating the nervous system which will have gone into sympathetic "fight or flight", and so welcoming a parasympathetic response that enables healing to land fully where is pain or dis-ease anywhere in the body is what I find working with 1M does.

I offer this as context for what I am about to share - just so that you can understand how much I love a high potency, and so how unusual it would be for me to say what I am about to share.

Most of the sacred geometry remedies are actually enough at 30c.

The vital force - the living weave of the microbiome and immune system with our soul; the expression of the ecosystem that we are - needs very little to find its harmony and balance once again. Giving really high potencies for most of the sacred geometry remedies can be a lot for many people - just as with other remedies. I use them generally as a support, in addition to other methods of prescribing - hence my offering of the *Blueprint Method,* which proposes the addition of these remedies as a support to heal and repair our Blueprint; our sacred geometry; the energetic fabric of who and what we are. Usually this does not require high potencies. Just like the microbiome doesn't usually need a massive blast of impetus to repair and heal itself, the same is true of our energy field, most of the time.

So I usually only work with 30c potencies for most of these remedies. They are powerful as they are, and can work and reach people in the most compromised of states.

Golden Spiral, in particular, given in high potency can trigger a strong detoxification response; it is a detoxifying remedy. It also reaches high into the spiral, rather than just giving enough of a catalyst at a lower potency from which the spiral can emerge to where it needs to be for the Vital Force to fully receive it.

Only occasionally where someone's energy is greatly compromised by the use of huge amounts of pharmaceuticals, drugs, or a highly toxic life, and the obstacles to cure or maintaining causes are great, and 30c doesn't reach what is needed, I may look to a 1M, but this is rare for me to do. There is an example of this in the 3rd case study listed in the Golden Spiral proving.

One exception to this is Metatron's Cube. Metrotron's Cube in higher potencies is beautiful for those whose Vital Force is able to receive high potencies well. It takes us to centre of creation; to life itself; the journey can be all the more beautiful in high potencies for those that can respond well to them. Dodecahedron can also be taken in higher potencies too.

Fibonacci Potencies

I would like to touch upon Fibonacci potencies (as single potencies only). I am often asked about why I talk about them only in standard potencies. I love the idea of Fibonacci potencies. I have tried some of the sacred geometry remedies in Fibonacci potencies however I have found that working with standard potencies seems to land better. I am not sure why, sometimes I wonder if it is perhaps because the consciousness of homeopathy is so deeply imprinted with the language of the standard potencies that our beings simply recognise and respond to them easily. I do love the idea in principle, but I have just found that standard potencies work so well.

Ascending Potencies

One of the ways of treating acutes or deeply entrenched conditions is using ascending potencies all in one day, from the lowest to the highest at regular intervals. For example taking one remedy in the next potency up every hour starting with 6x, then an hour later 6c, then another hour later 12c, and continuing with the next potency each other whilst working through 30c, 200c, 1M, 10M, 50M, CM, MM. As well as treating acutes without aggravations, prescribing in this way is like a reset – almost like the energetic equivalent of restarting the heart using a defibrillator, but more gentle. It also heals issues at a very deep level, and more deeply through time.

I find it to be a powerful way to work, but only in select situations, and when someone's Vital Force can receive it.

Giving an indicated sacred geometry remedy at the start of the day, along with the first potency can support and further deepen the clearing and healing. For example giving just one dose of Golden Spiral 30c at the start of the day can beautifully support and enhance the process.

Homochords

A final note on homochords (all potencies at the same time). This is different to Ascending Potencies all in one day. With Ascending Potencies all in one day, the Vital Force can receive the energetic vibration of that particular potency and process it before the next potency is introduced a little while later.

The sacred geometry remedies are not to be taken as homochords in any form. A homochord of these remedies will confuse the system. They are powerful energetically because they speak directly to our energy field, and so only a 'gentle nudge' to our energy field is needed in almost every case. They are powerful enough, even at a 30c. Homochords, especially of these remedies, risk overwhelming the system rather than supporting it.

The Golden Spiral Detox Protocol

I love working with detoxification protocols, especially Ton Jansen's protocols. I see such amazing results - I think some of my favourite work is detoxing synthetic hormones - from men as well as women. The level of empowerment I see in this is remarkable.

I completely understand the detoxification of the Covid-19 vaccines using the same tautopathic protocols, and completely respect this work being done by those who do so.

I just didn't, however, resonate with the vibration of the tautopathic remedies made from the Covid-19 vaccines. I tried really hard to become comfortable with them, but my whole being felt that I had found, for the first time, remedies I didn't feel I could give. So I invited guidance about what to use instead.

We didn't have Flower of Life back then, so the first blend I was intuitively guided to make was Golden Spiral, Thuja and Silica 30c. Two kinesiologists I didn't know, and who didn't know each other, independently contacted me in the same week, having heard of my protocol, and said they had tested it and it worked.

Since then, I have added Flower of Life, so the blend is:
Golden Spiral, Flower of Life, Thuja, Silica 30c

I still use tautopathy to detoxify every other drug, and then use this detox blend as the "Saturday Remedy" - Golden Spiral and Flower of Life are, after all, also organ support remedies.

However when detoxifying Covid-19 vaccines, I give this instead.

Protocol: one three times a day for 3-5 days then one daily for another 21 days.

I also recommend this to be taken daily during the week of flu vaccine spraying for those in school environments, or once a week just as a clearing for the body during flu spraying season.

The Golden Spiral Sarcodes

The Golden Spiral Sarcodes were developed as a result of working with two patients with very serious conditions, and I saw remarkable results. Since then, my favourite moment was seeing my then 15 year old son come home, two weeks after he had fractured his ankle (we saw the fracture on the x-ray), having worked with the ankle and foot sarcode, and he said "Mama, I've got something to show you", and then took his boot off, jumped up and down, and told me he'd been playing basketball. And he never felt any pain or discomfort with it again.

I was aware that organ support remedies came from human or animal sources, and we would never know the health or vitality of the donor. So I made them as a more detailed and comprehensive organ support, using the pure unconditional love of Source, asking for them to be made in a pure way. I have since evolved the series, and now there are over 40 Golden Spiral Sarcodes.

Each comprehensive sarcode is made up of all of the anatomical aspects of the relevant gland, hormone, organ or system, also including the blood vessels and nerves that supply it. The research to develop each Golden Spiral Sarcode has included anatomical information online, from detailed anatomical A&P books and information in the Sulis Database.

No radionics or other machines have been used in the making of these remedies: just a sacred space, altar and connection with the pure unconditional love of Source. All are made to a 1M potency unless otherwise stated (some hormone remedies are available in lower potencies).

In addition, each Golden Spiral Sarcode Blend contains:

Mastic Gum 1M
As made by me and proved by the Golden Spiral Provings Collective, a remedy that can act like a healing balm in the body, bringing repair where needed

Fasciae 1M
he fasciae hold any trauma or dysregulation, so releasing this may support the rebalancing of that gland, hormone, organ or system

Bosnian Pyramid of the Sun 30c
There are 18,000 negative ions per cubic cm within the tunnels (9 times more than is found within forests), and we found the remedy to be healing and regulating of all of the mind, body and spirit.

Golden Spiral 30c
The sacred geometry remedy for alignment, the vibrational sarcode of the DNA. Contains Phi mathematics; the vibration of love. The natural unfolding of life.

Flower of Life 30c
The sacred geometry for all of life and existence; the vibrational sarcode of the cell and the energy field. Contains Phi mathematics; the vibration of love.

Vector Equilibrium 30c
The sacred geometry remedy for a move from polarity to unity and peace

The following Blueprint Essence™

- Archangel Raphael (the Archangel of Healing)

Recommended dosage

During flare-ups or times of difficulty, one three times a day. Once the intensity has lessened or as low grade support, one daily.

Trademarks & Availability

These remedies speak to the blueprint of who and what we are. They are an expression of the vibration of love, truth & alignment.

I feel deeply privileged to be custodian of these remarkable remedies. I feel a deep responsibility to them and respect for the work they are here to do in this world.

Having a Trademark for each remedy protects the quality and purity of remedies, but also prevents confusion or a change to their vibration, and ensures that those who buy them are obtaining genuine remedies, made with integrity and love. I applied for trademarks not just for the names included here, but also any alternative similar names for each sacred geometry symbol.

The dispensaries that dispense these remedies do so with great care, integrity and alignment with love and respect for them. This ensures the exceptional quality of the remedies.

The trademarks apply to the production of single remedies, and also when used in combination with any other remedies, so they can only be sold by those licensed to do so.

An up-to-date list is available on my website of where the remedies can be obtained around the world.

Part 2

Sacred Geometry Remedies

The Golden Spiral

"[The universe] cannot be read until we have learnt the language and become familiar with the characters in which it is written. It is written in mathematical language, and the letters are triangles, circles and other geometrical figures, without which means it is humanly impossible to comprehend a single word."

- Galileo

About the Proving

This proving took place on 17th January 2021. 8 provers were involved in the first proving of this remedy. The 30c potency was used on this occasion by each prover.

The making of this remedy

This remedy was made on 21st December 2020, during the Winter Solstice, and the Great Jupiter-Saturn Conjunction that occurred on the same day. The Winter Solstice is the day when the Sun moves into Capricorn, and is the day in the year when we have the least number of daylight hours on the Earth. It is the shortest day, as it is the day in the year when the Earth is the furthest away from the Sun, and represents the end of darkness and a moving towards light.

The Jupiter-Saturn Conjunction is a special alignment of these two planets coming together (conjoining), which they do every 20 years. When they do so, they look like a single shining star in the sky from our vantage point.

In 1614, Johannes Kepler, a German mathematician and astronomer, theorised that the Star of Bethlehem, which showed the Three Wise Men (who were astrologers) where to find the baby Jesus, was a Saturn- Jupiter conjunction.[11] Before Kepler, there is a note of this in the Annals of the Abbey of Worcester dated 1285.[12]

The Jupiter-Saturn conjunction is said to show us where there are limitations, bringing in new ideas and creative thinking that can be used to solve old problems. In addition to this, there are new efforts for increased equality, freedom and respect, and an invitation to share our gifts and be more authentic.[13] All of this feels very relevant to
the Golden Spiral remedy, as does the fact that it was also made at the beginning of the Age of Aquarius.

The conjunction happened at 0 degrees of Aquarius – said to be the beginning of a 2,160 year era of community, sharing and working together.

The Winter Solstice, the Grand Conjunction and the dawning of the Age of Aquarius all symbolise new beginnings.

An essence was made by placing a vial of alcohol in an ancient oak tree in Greenwich Park, London, for safekeeping. This essence was then made into a remedy - the most vital version of the remedy was using the full Hahnemannian trituration method to a 12c before being made into higher potencies.

The intention had been to place the vial on the Meridian Line - the line where time starts counting around the world - however it was a blustery, stormy night and so my son climbed a little way up into an oak tree where there was a hollow that could look after the vial without it being blown away.

---

11 http://www.astronomynotes.com/history/bethlehem-star.html

12 https://astronomy.com/news/2020/12/the-star-of-bethlehem-can-science-explain-what-it-really-was

13 https://isarastrology.org/raymond-merriman-the-great-mutation-and-the-start-of-a-new-era-jupiter-and-saturn/

The vial remained there for 18 hours over the Solstice and Grand Conjunction. The vial was surrounded by pictures of the Golden Spiral, the numbers of the Fibonacci sequence which make up the Golden Spiral, and the number for Phi, symbolised by the Greek letter ϕ, which is also embodied in the Golden Spiral. The intention was set that the vial would capture the energy of all these. An intention was set that the tree would look after the vial without imprinting it's energies into the remedy - that it would be pure Golden Spiral that would be created.

The Golden Spiral

What is the Golden Spiral?

In order to understand the Golden Spiral, we need to remember the Fibonacci Sequence.

We return to an extract from *Nature's Medicine Code.*

As we have already seen, "we start at 0 and count up, each new number is the sum of the previous 2 numbers. So the sequence goes like this:

0+1 = 1
1+1 = 2
1+2 = 3
2+3 = 5
3+5 = 8
8+5 = 13
8+13 = 21

and so on, so the sequence looks like this:
0,1,1,2,3,5,8,13,21,34,55,89,144, 233......

If you divide one number in the Fibonacci sequence by the number before it, then you get Phi at any point from 89 onwards– or at the smaller numbers, a number very very very close to Phi. The further along the sequence you go, the closer and closer to the exact number of Phi you come……

When these numbers are drawn onto graph paper, with each number representing the size of the square a line is drawn in – so drawing across 1 square, then 1 square, then 2 squares, then 3, then 5, then 8 and so on carrying on using the Fibonacci sequence numbers, they form a pattern – it is a perfect ever growing spiral.

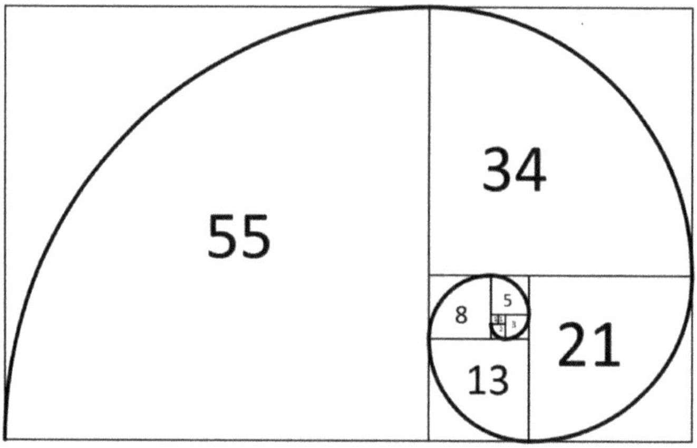

This spiral is called the Golden Spiral. It is a truly remarkable spiral, with the perfect geometric (mathematical) properties of Phi, and – according to Manfred Clynes – the vibration of love. This perfect mathematical spiral can be seen throughout nature, for example:

- In the famous nautilus
- In the proportions of our ears, how they grow and unfold
- The arrangement of faces, in particular the positioning of our mouth and nose along with our eyes and chin
- The proportions of the uterus
- In the spirals of the DNA
- In the growth and unfolding of leaves

- The number of petals a flower has
- The arrangement of seed heads, for example clearly seen in the sunflower
- The way in which branches on trees grow or split
- Animal bodies, including starfish, ants, honeybees, and the fins on dolphins
- How blood flows through blood vessels
- How hurricanes and tornados travel
- How currents flow in seas and oceans
- In the formation of ice crystals and snowflakes
- The Aurora Borealis (Northern Lights)
- How planets in our solar system orbit each other as they travel through the galaxy
- In how electrons flow around the nucleus of an atom[14]
- How the energy of balanced, healthy chakras flow
- How the soul enters and leaves the body

In fact, it has been proposed that phyllotaxis – the arrangement of leaves on a plant stem that follow the golden spiral – allows maximum levels of light capture, which maximises photosynthesis and plant growth. This was proposed by Strauss et al.[15]

In 2012, John J. Wille found that even single-celled prokaryotes, some of our smallest microorganisms contain Fibonacci patterns, as do motile (moving) single-celled bacteria that also organise themselves into "dynamic growth patterns resembling Fibonacci patterns".[16]

The Pyramids in Egypt also have the Golden Spiral geometry built

---

14 Winter, D, Donavan, B., and Jones, M. (2012) Compressions, The Hydrogen Atom and Phase Conjugation

15 Strauss, S et al., (2019) Phyllotaxis: is the golden angle optimal for light capture? New Phytologist (2020) 225:499-510

16 John J. Wille (2012) Occurrence of Fibonacci umbers in development and structure of animal forms: Phylogenetic observations and epigenetic significance Natural Science Vol 4, 216-232

into them, which suggests that they were designed in a very advanced way, and this geometry is found in the artwork of Michelangelo and Leonardo da Vinci. Some modern day artists and architects apply the principles of the Golden Spiral and the mathematics of Phi in their artistry and architectural design."

Dr Semir Osmaganich, who discovered the Bosnian Pyramids in Visoko, Bosnia in 2005 has been able to demonstrate how the Golden Spiral is found in the Bosnian Pyramid complex. The Bosnian Pyramids are aligned with the Pleiades star system. In 2025, Dr Osmaganich had his research into the Pleiades published, where he has mathematically proven that the Golden Spiral is found in the arrangement of some of the core stars that make up the Pleiades star system. [17]

The Fibonacci sequence has been found in the number of branches from vessels in the heart, and in the cardiac cycle of the human heart beat.[18]

There is one other way in which the Golden Spiral shows itself in life.

The Mandelbrot Set is a series of equations in Chaos Theory that measure the point at which order and chaos meet. When those equations are typed into computers a visual pattern – a fractal - is created.

The pattern is remarkable. If you zoom in to one part of the picture, you find the whole pattern from the bigger picture is repeated again within it. No matter how much you zoom in, you see the same pattern. The pattern unfolds using the geometry of the

---

17 Osmanagich, Sam. (2024). https://www.opastpublishers.com/open-access-articles/celestial-correspondence-and-geometric-patterning-the-pleiades-and-the-bosnian-valley-of-the-pyramids-9190.html. International Journal of Aerospace Science, Technology and Engineering. 1. 01-22. 10.33140/IJASTE.01.01.05.

18 Persaud-Sharma D and O'Leary JP. Fibonacci Series, Golden Proportions, and the Human Biology. Auln J Surg. 2015; 2 (5): 1066

Golden Spiral. It basically shows the continual unfolding of life; how the macrocosm is a reflection of the microcosm and vice versa in a continual unfolding of the spiral through life.

It is a reminder of the importance of both order and chaos in order to allow the spiral of life to unfurl; too much order (suppression), and the spiral of life can't emerge. Too much chaos and it becomes unstable. But a balance of both allows the perfect expression and natural expansion that life wishes to experience.

Another great example of the Mandelbrot set can be found in the maps of the body found in the hands, feet, eyes and ears. We have a whole human body, but reflexologists massage smaller versions those same parts of the whole human body through the map of the body found represented on the hands and the feet.

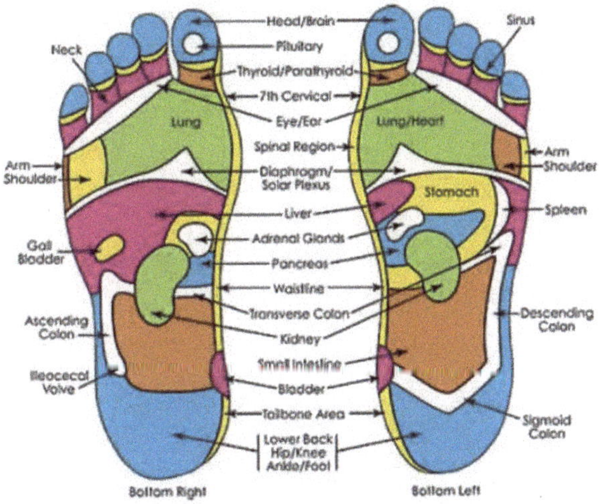

Iridologists can see what is happening in the body through the map of the body made miniscule in the eyes. Oricular acupuncturists treat people using the map of the body made smaller and found in the ears.

I would also suggest that the Mandelbrot Set is a visual representation of the Doctrine of Signatures! Trees, which are crucial for the gaseous exchange of carbon dioxide for oxygen, are a much larger version of our own human lungs. The tree trunk looks like the trachea, with the larger branches like bronchi, smaller branches like bronchioles and leaves where gaseous exchange occurs like our alveoli, where gaseous exchange happens within our bodies.

As well as helping to prevent cancer, The New Scientist reported the work of Shyam Biswal and her colleagues at John Hopkins University[19] who found that broccoli may also help the immune system to clean harmful bacteria from the lungs. A compound found in the vegetable is now being trialled as a treatment for people with lung disease. Broccoli also looks like a mini tree, and is an example of how this repeating pattern is expressed in food we put into our bodies. Walnuts look like the brains they nourish, kidney beans look like the kidneys they nourish too.

The Mandelbrot Set is an expression of the Golden Spiral, which contains within it the key number Phi.

It feels important to mention the work of Dr Masuro Emoto (1943 – 2014). He was a Japanese scientist who devoted the later years of his life to taking microscopic photos of ice crystals that form when water from different sources is frozen. Pure unpolluted water, when frozen, produces the most perfect stunningly beautiful water crystals – snowflakes – with perfect geometric Phi patterns. Polluted water, when frozen, produces completely malformed crystals, with no geometry, no clear patterns,
and have no clear form or shape to them.

He took photographs of ice crystals formed from ordinary water that

19 https://www.newscientist.com/ar1cle/dn20378-broccoli-helps-clear-damaged-lungs/

has been sat in a glass jug over a piece of paper with the word "love" on it. And then water that has been sat on the word "hate". Water that just sits on the word "love" produces perfect and stunningly beautiful ice crystals, and water sitting on the word hate freezes in the same malformed way as polluted water.

The ice crystals – snowflakes – of pure water, or water that is connected with love have a perfect hexagonal geometry that contains within it Phi (1.618), which Manfred Clynes measured to be the frequency of love, as well as the geometry of the Golden Spiral. This is missing from the crystals formed from polluted or hate-filled water.

Dr Emoto also took photos and made videos of what happened when music was played to those ice crystals. Harmonious music (such as classical music) would cause the perfectly geometrical ice crystals to unfold like petals of a flower opening.

Disharmonious sound vibrations would cause the ice crystals to lose their geometric properties. This makes sense in the context of Pythagoras' work, who, by adding in the musical 5th, which we described at the beginning of this journey into The Golden Spiral and Phi mathematics. Pythagoras' discovery of adding the extra note to the 7 note musical scale to create an octave brought in the number Phi (love) to music and was able to generate *harmonia;* harmony. Videos such as the one referenced here show this remarkable effect.[20]

So the Golden Spiral is a mathematical and geometric expression of love, the natural world, health, in Pythagoras' words *harmonia* – and life itself.

20 https://www.youtube.com/watch?v=gVbhSvT9-Fk

Golden Spiral Homeopathic Remedy™

Key Themes

Alignment & Flow
Expansion
Purpose
Peace, Stillness, Calm, Acceptance & Trust
Strength & Resilience
Connection
Truth
Freedom from Limitations & Constraints
Transitions
DNA repair
Energy giving
Sound
WW2

Alignment & Flow

One of the greatest aspects of this remedy is that it is a remedy that brings alignment in all it's forms; at a cellular level including in the DNA, structurally within the body including with the skeletal system, emotionally and with our thinking so that we can align ourselves with decisions and actions that connect us with our purpose. The Golden Spiral is the expression of alignment, flow, growth, and expansion. The remedy spirals through us, finding the ways in which our natural state of flow, growth and expansion are blocked, stuck or stagnant, and clears these, so that the spiral can be in alignment again; so that we can flow.

So this remedy finishes off past unfinished healing processes. This remedy clears old shadows, heals old traumas, pain and hurts that still haven't yet been healed, even where a person has done a lot of work on the issue or the pain. This remedy moves emotions outwards in a spiral. It seems to go "back" in time to seek what needs to be healed before moving "forward" to clear the way ahead.

As one prover said "I found myself revisiting the past, needing to go back to the past to where I chose a path that wasn't up to my potential – I was taken back to that choice. It's like I was going back to remember who I was in order to be able to move forward".

As well as reconnecting us with past situations, the Golden Spiral can take us back to past relationships that we have lost touch with that are meaningful at a deeper soul level, even if in a dream state, bringing healing to these.

The Golden Spiral also reconnects us with the totality of who we are; an alignment with mind, body, soul & spirit using Goethe's model. The Golden Spiral brings us back into integrity in all ways; mentally, emotionally, physically and spiritually; it helps to close the gap where dis-ease may have set in.

Where there is a misalignment physically, particularly with the spine, it might not necessarily align the posture, but it will align the connections through the spine.

Interestingly, when we look at the skeletal system, with the skull at the top branching down into ever smaller bones down our body, it could be said to be like a giant tuning fork. It's crystalline nature means that it is a great conductor of energy, and it is said by some ancient wisdoms to be a giant tuning fork for the energy of the Universe. If this is the case, a misalignment in our spine or skeletal system can make it difficult to receive a healthy and uninterrupted flow of energy through it, and it is this that the Golden Spiral remedy helps to resolve.

The alignment that the Golden Spiral brings can be about who we are. This remedy invites us to be completely aligned with our authentic selves. Like Thuja, this remedy is revealing, but also the Golden Spiral spirals out the energy of what has been revealed in order to enable the individual to move forward.

One of the provers was reminded of the actor Robert de Niro, who spent many years playing Mafioso / gangster type roles. He has since expanded out of his stereotype, into the fullness of who he can be as an actor........playing a man with an extreme form of locked in catatonia and the late stages of a Parkinson's-like illness in *Awakenings* in which he co-starred with Robin Williams. In the film *Stardust,* his character surprises us with a wonderful twist as a trans pirate. Robert de Niro has expanded beyond the perceived character limitations his early roles might have created into the fullness of all he can be as an actor. In a similar way, the Golden Spiral provides the energy to enable us to step out of stereotypes and limitations, so that we can be all of who we really are, and who we are capable of being. This remedy enables us to step into a much greater role, into much greater possibilities.

Another aspect of alignment, is that when we feel aligned with ourselves, we have the strength to make choices that support that.

Another film analogy shared by one of the provers came from *Star Wars.* In the final trilogy, the man character Rey, who has been fighting on the side of the Rebellion (the "goodies" in the films), discovers that she is the granddaughter of the evil Emperor (the supreme "baddie" in the films). The focus in the films is her journey, and the choices she makes, which are about choosing to be a Jedi using "The Force" for good, focusing on the Light despite her background, being fully aligned to herself and to something greater.

In a similar way, this remedy facilitates strong choices, based on our truth and what resonates with us, once we are aligned.

In bringing us into alignment, this remedy also is a remedy that is useful for those who feel ungrounded, as it is very grounding. It aligns us with the Earth as much as it does the Heavens, and with ourselves and where we are. (Oak, Thuja).

The Golden Spiral brings alignment where there is a dichotomy or binary experience – it brings us back to centre; to a singularity. Where there is division, or a "black and white" polarity, this remedy unites us and brings us together, which correlates with Pythagoras' *harmonia.* This remedy brings harmony and balance.

One prover described coming back to "a completely beingness, a complete alignment. Anything where there is a divide, or a two or a polarity doesn't need to be there anymore. We've seen in the past few years that this binary is so damaging. We are living through the era of that – left/right, leave/remain, Tory/Labour, whatever the binary is....it's not helping us in any way". This is a remedy that brings us back to Oneness; to a state of centre and a state of balance. In this alignment we find peace.
Once we are aligned, it is easier to manifest too. This remedy can be a tool for manifesting that which is aligned with our path. Dreams will be unfulfilled if we are unaligned; we cannot receive the energy or flow to make them happen. The Golden Spiral aligns us so that we can connect with those dreams again and manifest more easily what is aligned for us to manifest.

Expansion

The theme of expansion is of great significance with this remedy; there is an opportunity to expand beyond current limitations. The Golden Spiral gives energy for this to occur. Doors can open that we didn't know were there.

One prover gave this description:
"The metaphor that I got was that of an eggshell. With an eggshell

what you've got inside is the membrane, and inside that is the baby bird. What I got from this was that, the person or bird can be encapsulated in something. That's their world, that's all they know, they don't know anything outside of that. They wouldn't even begin to understand out in the garden, let alone out in space – it doesn't know what it doesn't
know. The remedy I felt was an interface, a bit like the membrane would be for the bird. So the bird has got to break out of this membrane, out into the shell, or the bird (or person or we) can choose to look inwards and look to do the work ourselves.

I feel that what the remedy does is it is a pull – it can go either way – and particularly as practitioners, it can give capabilities to patients to do this themselves. You could use this for patients with locked-in syndrome, in deep catatonic states, in deep depressions.....those people who are locked in, in their own emotional state. It will give them a way to be able to find a way out. Not necessarily guided by you or by someone else, but their own cells and soul within trying to find a solution trying to bring them out of that."

We are living in a time of expansion; "new ways of banking, new ways of health, new ways of looking at drugs, new ways of countries working together, new ways of interplanetary connection", as was described in the proving. This remedy aligns us with expansion in ways that are a reflection of – or a return to – the expression of love, as embodied in the mathematics of Phi.

We also need the *freedom* to expand, so freedom is inherent in this remedy. In this way it can be quite a Tubercular remedy.

Purpose

The Golden Spiral aligns us with our purpose. As human beings, we can at times veer off wildly in directions that aren't in alignment with who we are, or our purpose. The analogy of trying to keep humans on their paths being like having to herd cats sprung to mind. We can be so afraid of expanding into the fullness of who and what we can be, and can make all sorts of excuses and create all sorts of distractions to avoid living our greatest lives. This remedy is a cat (human) herder; it brings us back into alignment with our purpose.

Where we have strayed away from our life path because of fear, the Golden Spiral brings with it feelings of safety and protection, strength and a feeling of being able to move forward.

As Joseph Campbell said " We must let go of the life we have planned, so as to accept the one that is waiting for us".

This remedy quietens aspects of the ego that may have gone out of balance, so that we can realign with purpose in this way. And in so doing, as one prover described: "almost like this giant amongst whatever little challenges there might be, that might been big on a human level, but actually once I've stepped into that space, they feel tiny".

Another prover described feeling like "an unstoppable force for love and for goodness and like I could do ANYTHING".

The Golden Spiral reconnects us with an inner strength, and inspires self-sufficiency; a self-reliance, a knowing of what needs to be done, without the same previous need for external help.

This remedy has a very strong relationship with Lycopodium - it's all about expanding into your fullness and who you are; growing into yourself.

Peace, Stillness, Calm, Acceptance & Trust

The Golden Spiral brings with it these feelings of peace, stillness, calm and
acceptance; a tranquillity and trust that all is as it is meant to be.

One prover described it in this way about a headache she was experiencing. "Even though there's a physical pain there.....there is also an acceptance of whatever I was in physically, mentally, emotionally, spiritually".

The absolute stillness and calm was experienced within the person, and spiralling out externally. The peace and acceptance that the Golden Spiral brings is similar to Lotus.

These feelings also made it easier to breathe. Where the Epstein-Barr virus proving found that it helped with the inbreath, this remedy facilitates the outbreath; a letting go, a peace and calm.

Even where there is a lot of grief or anger or sadness, this remedy lightens these, or brings a sense of peace even when feeling these emotions. It brings an acceptance of challenges, even if the situation hasn't changed. The Golden Spiral helps us to feel differently about those situations, and lifts us out of the pain so that we can see them in a new way.

Because the Golden Spiral goes "back" into the issue before moving it forward, it can help us to see what the issue is that is causing the problems. It helps us to identify the emotions behind the issue, bringing a sense of peace in acknowledging what they are. As one prover described, the Golden Spiral "brings up lost secrets from the depths of the soul". This remedy then opens and dissipates these out from the centre of the spiral, releasing them.

With this comes a feeling of being lifted emotionally, emotional issues don't feel as heavy, and a strong sense of trust. The trust is in knowing that you are on the right path, a trust in your ability to move forward, a trust in intuition, and that there has been an alleviation of constraints.

This remedy may be useful as an escort for inner journeys, for example in isolation tanks, hypnosis and regression work.

In spiralling out uncomfortable emotions, the Golden Spiral then opens us up to hope, happiness, laughter, lightness, positivity and joy.

With it can come an optimism, a hope for change, and an excitement and a desire to connect, and to do new things. Almost like a sense of a spring clean – a complete emotional, physical, energetic spring clean.

Strength & Resilience

The Golden Spiral brings with it a renewed strength and resilience. The energy of moving forward in alignment with yourself and your purpose requires inner strength to take actions that maintain that alignment. This may include having the strength to speak up or make decisions in situations that it might have been difficult to do so previously.

It may be easier to draw healthy boundaries without worrying about the consequences in the same way (Carcinosin, Blue, Blackbird, Emerald). This remedy brings a greater ability to recognise what resonates and doesn't resonate, which makes us stronger in ourselves. This awareness gives us a greater choice as to how we move forward.

This remedy brings not just a greater emotional strength, but also a physical one.

Provers reported feeling strong physically – robust, resilient, undefeatable, indestructible. There can be a greater feeling of safety, of feeling protected (Vernix).

Connection

Another aspect of alignment that this remedy helps with is connection – to who we really are, to peace, acceptance, purpose, to our life path, to core relationships, to all we need to live, "to the flow of all life that wants to express itself through you", as one prover described; the "ultimate connection remedy".

In the running up of the remedy, there was a sense of a huge expansive energy, with light expanding through the room, and the entire building, connecting with a Higher self, and with a Higher aspect (Source or God, if you will). The prover who ran the remedy up wrote at one point "God molecule"; referring to the pure unconditional love of Source, or whatever we call that energy. Dr Hahnemann's "Spirit".

This connection to Source came up several times during the running of the remedy and in the proving, as did a connection not just to ourselves and our life paths, but also to the Universe / Cosmos, including a connection with the angels, and other aspects of us in other lifetimes and realities.

This is consistent with the Mandelbrot set fractals which show how everything is connected.

Truth

The Golden Spiral is a big truth remedy, aligning us with our truth. It enables us feel what does and doesn't resonate, and this in part is what makes us stronger and more resilient.

Feeling connected with ourselves, we are able to speak our truth.

Part of how this remedy brings acceptance is by inviting you to accept the truth of
things and how they are. As one prover said "What we see may not be pretty but this remedy helps us to accept the truth of things and how they are". This is another way in which this remedy is revealing (Thuja).

Freedom from Limitations & Constraints

The Golden Spiral is an expression of the natural flow of energy and life. Wherever there are blocks and limitations, this remedy clears these, to make way for this natural flow of life.

The remedy brings "this incredible freedom, this alleviation from constraints; a release" as one prover described. "Almost like a miasmatic feeling of constraint and then release".

Those constraints can be physical, mental, emotional or spiritual, and may even go through time. As we will see shortly, there was a strong connection to WW2 during the proving, and this remedy brought a freedom from constraints experienced then. As one prover described it, "dark forces being alleviated". This remedy was described during the proving as a remedy "to bring the end of all darkness and the end of all
wars".

There is an empowerment aspect to this remedy; where the

limitations or constraints have been by leaders being controlling or dictatorial in any way; this remedy moves us towards a greater freedom. We found that this can even be applied to limitations in our thinking; not believing in our own ability to heal ourselves for example. This remedy moves us beyond these limiting thoughts to possibilities and being more in our own power to effect positive changes.

Transitions

The Golden Spiral clears blockages, fears, and limitations so that we can move forward in a way that is aligned. This remedy, therefore, helps with transitions; with moving from one state or place in time, from unhealthy situations, into healthy ones.

This remedy is useful wherever there is any resistance to a transition, or fear of the unknown. It may also be useful during life transitions that are challenging or changeable such as adolescence and menopause.

The Golden Spiral may also be useful as an end-of-life remedy, particularly where someone is finding it difficult to let go. All energy, all of natural life, spirals out using this mathematics and geometry, and so may help the soul to pass using natural energy cycles found in all of life.

DNA repair

One of the most important themes for this remedy is the work it does with the DNA.

The Golden Spiral, as we have seen, is reflected in the mathematical and geometric properties of the DNA.

Where this has been damaged or compromised in any way, this remedy reminds the DNA of its true structure and nature.

The Golden Spiral brings alignment to the DNA, strengthens and activates it. It works within our DNA to repair our cells; it helps us to heal our own cells. This remedy gives energy to the DNA strands spiralling up, spinning upwards, and activates them. This remedy helps the DNA to "come alive" as one prover described, strengthening the life force. This remedy helps all our cells to vibrate with life.

Energy giving

Mitochondria are the organelles within a cell that generate adenosine triphosphate (ATP) – energy. They are in fact, according to Dr Zach Bush, part of our microbiome; of bacterial origin. He states; "They can replicate and reproduce within our cells. They can die within our cells independent of the survival of our cells. The typical human cell has approximately 200 mitochondria per cell, which is different than you see in a biology textbook that traditionally only shows you two. Longevity of the cell is now recognised to have a lot to do with the health and number of the mitochondria within it.

Some of the nutrients will get absorbed into a cell, and consumed by the mitochondria.[21] They are consumed through the citric acid/Krebs cycle, and the respiratory chain. During this process, they are delivering electrons to the respiratory chain, a chain of enzymes in the wall of the mitochondria, converting adenosine diphosphate to adenosine triphosphate."[22]

---

21 Madeira VMC. Overview of mitochondrial bioenergelcs

22 https://www.liebertpub.com/doi/full/10.1089/act.2019.29220.zbu

Our cells are full of these 'bugs', or mitochondria, and these little microorganisms are feeding us. When we eat, the nutrients from the food have to go through the digestive tract, where they are first exposed to bacteria or fungi, and then the breakdown products or metabolites of microbial activity are absorbed by our body. The nutrients get repackaged in complex structures by the liver and then sent back out into the periphery, eventually ending up in our cells. We know that bacteria contain Fibonacci patterns, so it makes sense that Phi mathemaıcs and geometry would also be found in mitochondria, which are bacterial in origin.

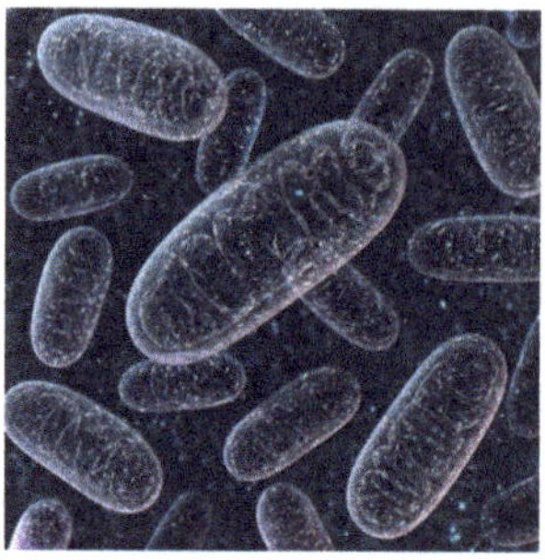

At the time of writing, a study where this has been measured could not be found, but we understood in the proving that there is a relationship between the mitochondria, the Golden Spiral mathematics and geometry, and the mitochondria's ability to generate ATP (energy).

This remedy helps with the mitochondria's ability to generate ATP – so it has a big connection with fatigue. One prover said "This is an energy-giving, life force giving remedy. It's a direct connection to the vital force".

ATP cannot be generated when the liver is sluggish. What this remedy does is it works on both levels – it helps detoxify, almost like a Carduus Marianus (Milk Thistle) action with the liver, and yet at the

same time it helps the mitochondria to do what they need to generate ATP.
Antibiotics damage mitochondria, which make sense given their bacterial origins.[23]

Glyphosate is an antibiotic as well as a weedkiller (herbicide), so foods that contain glyphosate can damage the mitochondria and so affect our energy levels. All foods that are not organic contain glyphosate. Even then, some organic crops have been affected by spraying in neighbouring farms. Kate Birch's essay on glyphosate and it's actions on the body have been detailed in her book *Glyphosate Free.*[24]

There is a symbiotic relationship between humans and bacteria and viruses. We need naturally occurring viruses, bacteria and fungi as part of our evolution, and to maintain our health. The balance of these are damaged by antibiotic use, and also
the use of chemical sterilisers and sanitisers.

During the proving, we were shown that the Golden Spiral remedy directly restores a balance between the different aspects of the human ecosystem; with the virome and the biome and with fungi. It can help in balancing out some of the damage done to the ecosystem through our use of these drugs and chemicals.

This remedy brings peace and calm not just to us, but to the bacteria and other microbes that are part of our ecosystem, where they are out of balance. In the same way that it brings harmony and balance to our human relationships, or the relationship between paired organs, it also brings healing to the relationships within our ecosystem; between us, the bacteria, viruses and fungi that maintain and support our health.

---

23 https://pubmed.ncbi.nlm.nih.gov/23825301/
24 Kate Birch (2019) Glyphosate Free. Kate Birch

The Golden Spiral remedy helps old trapped, stagnant energy to be released. This is a very important remedy for the liver. It helps to clear things out, it helps to release toxicity, enables healthy movement and flow.

It may also be that the mitochondria are evolving as our bodies are vibrating faster, and we are generating higher frequencies of energy. The Golden Spiral may also support mitochondria and other parts of us with the generation of photons and light energy too.

Sound

This remedy heightened the hearing of several provers. This aligns with how the Golden Spiral and Phi mathematics is also found in harmonious music, and there is a strong connection between sound and the Golden Spiral.

Some of the sounds that were heard more clearly were physical sounds, others were more the ability to hear the heartbeat of the Earth (the Schumann Resonances).

World War 2

Nearly half of the provers described some connection to WW2. We are still living with the effects of WW2 in many ways. Epigenetically, many of us will carry the impact of the World Wars, the trauma of which will have passed down through our DNA. Many of us may have had an experience of being involved at that time; of having had a lifetime there.

The Golden Spiral goes back to that time and releases unhealed trauma that may have passed down epigenetically, or have happened in another lifetime. This is a remedy that reaches far back in time. We connected specifically with WW2, but feel that this is a remedy for any war trauma, particularly if it goes far back (Berlin Wall, Japanese White Oleander). This includes WW1 and the Russian Revolution. It is a remedy that brings healing to darker times and experiences in the past.

These experiences, all have something in common. They don't have the laws of nature and love flowing through them, and their effects have been devastating. This remedy clears the effect of these events that may have thrown us out of alignment. We become aligned again.

Mental & Emotional Symptoms

Deep depression
Depression with loss of body movement or catatonia
Dark depression - cannot see a way out (Aurum). This remedy helps give a way out
Feeling of being held captive, physical or imagined
Sadness
Melancholy
Unhealed trauma from the past
Deep grief
Feeling of loss of freedom (real or imagined)
A need to speak out
A sudden desire to run a mile, to start moving, to start dancing
Lack of purpose
Loss of direction or meaning in life
Feeling stuck
Unable to move forward
Difficulty making decisions

Physical Particulars

Head

Pressure above head
Brain fog / fuzziness
Fizzing in the head
Headache moving between eyeball and back of the head to top of head, might move
down to back of the neck
Band around the head
Tight sensation, like being squeezed, around the whole head
Tight sensation around the temples
Tight sensation in the front of the head
Tight sensation in the head, moving down to the occiput
Ocular migraine
Sinus pressure – upper sinuses, moving into the head
Sinusitis
Feeling off balance / off centre
Vertigo, worse when opens eyes
Head feeling blocked
Bones in head – if out of alignment
Pain in facial bones or skull
Dyslexia

Eyes

Photophobia, especially in right eye
Yellow eyes
Ears
Blocked ears
High pitched "eeeeeeeee" sound in ears
Loss of balance
Car sickness
Hearing heartbeat in ears (from fear)

Nose

Blocked nose – thick coryza
Sinus pressure – upper sinuses, moving into the head
Sinusitis
Blocked sinuses
Sensitivity to exhaust fumes and other toxins

Mouth & Teeth

Burning lips
Throbbing in the gums in the front teeth
Misaligned teeth that cause an imbalance in the relevant Traditional Chinese
Medicine (TCM) organ, according to the TCM chart

Neck

Tension in neck and shoulders

Throat

Swollen glands
Difficulty swallowing
Catarrh – needing to clear from the throat
Clearing congestion
Fuzzy feeling in throat
Fizzing in the throat

Lungs

Those who have used a respirator, to re-connect with natural rhythms of breathing in
and out

Shallow breathing
Fuzzy feeling in lungs
Fizzing in the lungs

Heart

Elevated heartrate
Hearing heartbeat in ears (from fear)
Arrhythmia
Atrial fibrillation

Liver

Sluggish liver
Fatigue
Toxicity
Cirrhosis of the liver
Yellow skin (jaundice)
Yellow eyes
Cholestasis
Jaundice

Kidneys, Bladder, Urination

Frequency of urination
Incomplete urination
Poor kidney function
Fizzing in the bladder
Pain in one or both kidneys
Dull ache in one or both kidneys

Digestion

Dysbiosis
Borborygmi

Trapped flatus
Yellow stools
Greasy stools
Gall bladder pain
Constipation
Bloating

Back & Limbs

Still joints, where a release is needed, better movement
Stiff back, where a release is needed, better movement
Rigidity in limbs
Crack in skin on big toe
Cracked hands or feet
Blue hands or feet
Hands and feet cannot get warm when cold
Poor circulation to hands and feet
Swollen hands and arms, up to elbow
Heavy calves
Skin
Crack in skin on big toe
Cracked hands or feet
Blue hands or feet
Blue skin
Yellow skin
Inflamed (red) skin

Physical Generals

Body Temperature
Chilly body states – extremes out of alignment
Hot body states – extremes out of alignment

Food & Thirst

Poor assimilation of nutrients
Dreams
Dreams of war, especially previous World Wars

Bodily fluids

Lymph nodes affected as if coming up to something like a cold
Energy
Low vital force
Fatigue
Exhaustion

Clinical

Cancer - all cancers
Parkinson's Disease
Locked in states
Neurological damage
Multiple sclerosis
Dopamine imbalance
Cholestasis
Mast Cell Activation
Arrhythmia
Atrial fibrillation
Any condition where one of a paired organ is functioning less well than the other part of the pair

Modalities

Better movement
Better fresh air
Better warmth
Better sunshine

Better for being in nature

Sensations

Tight sensation around the forehead as if the skull was being squeezed
A warm sensation throughout whole body, as if held by another
Fuzzy head, as if off centre
Tenderness of joints where the different parts of the skull come together at the vertex, as if I had had an osteopathic treatment
Throbbing in the gums in the front four teeth, as if I was a rabbit
Sensation of lungs being ventilated, as if there was an automatic breathing occurring
Lymph nodes affected as if a cold is coming on

Spiritual

The Golden Spiral is helpful for practitioners, lightworkers, soul people that have obviously come into this life to experience things and learn things and use the skills that we've had from other lifetimes on the Earth or on other planets, making it easier to work on ourselves as we and the planet evolve.

This remedy connects us to Source, to ourselves and our life paths, but also spiritually to the Universe / Cosmos, including a connection with the angels, and other aspects of us in other lifetimes and realities. It connects us with a wide range of vibrations,
which may be seen as colours or heard as sounds.

We were shown that the flow of energy of the angels also is in this Golden Spiral geometry and mathematics – that all energy that supports life, health, love, connection and happiness does.

It's a very light remedy; there is lots of light that comes in through it.

It activates the pineal gland.

Where the aura needs repairing, because it has become tired, or damaged, or unhealthy looking, with holes in it, looking at all moth eaten, or it has any shade of brown or any sooty texture, the Golden Spiral works to repair the aura. This remedy does the equivalent of shaking out a duvet, clearing out all of the dust and the debris, so that the whole energy field becomes pure and white and glistening and shining, vibrating and radiating.

Vibration is really important with this remedy. This remedy raises the vibration of the energy field of those who take it. One prover described feeling "electrically charged".

It also aligns the chakras so that they flow in a balanced way. Each chakra ideally oscillates or spirals in the opposite direction to the chakra on either side of it; the chakras alternating between clockwise and anticlockwise flows of energy. Flowing in these ways generates a vortex, and a spiral between the chakras, which gives us strength. The vortex enables the whole of the energy field to flow properly.

Microwave energy, including 5G radiation, can affect these oscillations, and send the chakras out of balance. Also any genetic modification can lead to a collapse of one of more of the chakras, which in turn leads to an energetic disconnection from all that the chakras connect us with. This remedy may help the DNA to remember and reconnect with it's natural structure, mathematics and geometry.

The Golden Spiral remedy was experienced by one prover as spiralling all the way from the DNA, right up into the cosmos – like in the Mandelbrot fractal patterns, that describe the holographic nature of the Universe.

We have been taught that we have 7 core chakras, with more chakras beyond these 7. I teach that we have 8 core chakras based on Phi mathematics. Pythagoras, the Ancient Greek mathematician, astrologer, astronomer, scientist and musician, found that, when he played a string instrument called a lyre, that he could create a perfect *harmonia* if he added a sharp half-note to a 7 note musical scale. This extra note – called the "musical fifth" sits after the 4th note in a 7 note scale, and its addition creates what Pythagoras named an octave.

There is a mathematical ratio found between the 4th and 5th notes in an octave – Phi (1.618) – the number for love as we explored earlier. If we apply this model to the chakras, and add in a small chakra after the 4th......it gives us the Thymus Gland chakra, and brings an octave, or *harmonia* to our energy. That's when you get perfect balance. Adding in this chakra, which connects us with our immune system in the physical body, and with the timeline through which all of our experiences in every lifetime are recorded, brings true alignment.

The Golden Spiral remedy might be a wonderful aid to take just before meditations.

This is hugely karmic remedy, working through time.

It is also a Blueprint remedy; a remedy that connects with who we are, and can be used alongside the Triad method where there is an organ support at the bottom, then fundamental/lesion layer, then a miasmatic remedy at the top of the Triad. Blueprint remedies sit above these layers, connecting us with our Blueprint, or soul. The Blueprint Method encompasses all of these.

This is a remedy that helps us move from the 3D into the 5D; it is an Ascension remedy.

Chakras

Soul star

The Golden Spiral remedy connects us with the highest possibility that we've got – higher than we would normally consider, higher than the crown chakra – it just goes beyond. With our awareness we can open more crown chakras, as far as we feel able to go.

Crown

Several provers reported a strong sensation, or pressure above the physical head, in the Crown. Each reported the pressure feeling positive, as though "a Higher Source was there, very loving, very supportive". All of the chakras being aligned is important with this remedy, and is part of the healing of the remedy. Once the remedy has balanced the other chakras, the Crown can open to progress to a higher awareness spiritually; a transformation.

A lack of consciousness or in catatonic patients, the Crown can be totally closed; just their physical bodies are working. This remedy can support the opening of the Crown chakra.

This remedy can help people pass over and transition also, through the Crown. It brings peace, inviting the questions "where am I supposed to be right now? Is it on the Earth or is it elsewhere?", so that the person can align with where their soul chooses to be, and helps them to move towards it. It may help support the soul's move through any drugs that they may be taking also.

Third Eye

The Golden Spiral invites us to take responsibility for our own health and look inwards to our health and our own physical repairing, and this is seen at the Third Eye chakra; using our intuitive senses to look into ourselves, and identify what we need to do to repair what in need of repair. This remedy gives us the opportunity to see more about what we can do, rather than looking outwards expecting everybody else to fix everything for us, if we would choose that.

This remedy also helps connect us to our Blueprint though this chakra.

Throat

The Golden Spiral gives us the energy to speak our truth with love, honouring our boundaries. It unblocks stagnant energy at this chakra. It also helps us to accept ourselves and feel peace when we have spoken our truth to others, even if it may have been challenging to do so, feeling free from being affected by any criticisms from others in doing so because of being in complete alignment with ad in integrity with oneself (Carcinosin, Blackbird). This remedy brings a tremendous feeling of calm in having done so.

Higher Heart (Thymus Chakra)

This chakra is the point of connection and disconnection physically (with our health), and through time with ourselves in all lifetimes. The Golden Spiral reconnects us where we may be disconnected. This remedy works through all of our lifetimes, bringing alignment through time and space. It may appear as rainbow coloured following the taking of this remedy.

Heart

This remedy brings feelings of the heart expanding, peace, stillness, calm. The Golden Spiral embodies love, and it spirals (radiates) love outwards, but also perhaps more importantly, inwards. Self-love is still something that many find hard to do, and this remedy helps with that. It reveals what we may need so that we can fully align

(Thuja, Carcinosin, Rainbow).

There may also be feelings of warmth and lightness – almost as though the Sun is shining in through the heart, helping it heal.

This remedy connects us with what is possible – endless possibilities, once we are aligned and love ourselves enough to open to them.

Solar plexus

This remedy brings a feeling of being really centred, and aligned with our truth. We know what feels right based on our gut feeling – It's our solar plexus that tells us what resonates and what doesn't resonate - what feels right and what doesn't' feel right, we feel it right there. So the Golden Spiral connects us with our gut feelings so we can
discern what feels true for us and what doesn't and to let that go without judgement.

Sacral

This chakra is all about relationships with others. This remedy is all about our relationship with ourselves. It brings healing to past and current relationships through healing the relationship with the self, and bringing in feelings of peace there. This remedy aligns the chakras, however, not so we can focus on others, but so we can be aligned with ourselves and move forward strongly on that basis. As one prover said, "you do you".

Creativity comes into this chakra too. This remedy brings flowerings of creativity, helps us to connect with old and new ways of expressing our creativity, and recognises the importance of doing so.

Root

The Root is where much of the trauma people experience is held – people's root chakras can literally be shattered. This is a useful to take alongside root chakra remedies to help to clear those traumas. The Root still holding trauma makes it difficult for the person to be in alignment, so this work is hugely important, as being able to ground fully facilitates expansion.

The more that we are grounded, the higher our energy can travel too through the Crown chakra. You need to feel secure to be able to explore inwards and look at shadow, but also to expand into the fullness of who you are and who you are here to be.

The trauma that happens to this chakra in this world can create a binary effect, which means people can't fully ground properly and can't be fully whole and this remedy moves from a binary state to a singularity at the root, and in fact it does that with all of the chakras – wherever there is a binary state, there will be just a singularity going forward.

It is a grounding remedy, like Oak, Thuja & T-Rex.

Earth Star

The Golden Spiral will likely be found in the remarkable mycelial network, which are all those threads under the ground. We used to think it was just mud, and now we realise there are trillions and trillions of organisms, and this is the chakra through which, when healed, that we are literally joined with everything else on the Earth. We are made of fungus as well. We connect with breathing organisms down into the Earth. deeper you go into the Earth, the more you connect with other people. Living breathing organisms and Gaia. Crystals will also contain the geometry of the Golden Spiral and Fibonacci mathematics, and this remedy reconnects with the Oneness we have with Earth when we are aligned.

Remedy Affinities

Ayahuasca (karmic clearing)
Berlin Wall (war trauma)
Blackbird (Speaking up, with love)
Blue (Speaking up)
Carcinosin (revealing, drawing boundaries once aligned with oneself and one's truth)
Emerald (drawing healthy boundaries, radiation)
Japanese White Oleander (war trauma)
Lanthanides series (freedom)
Lotus (stillness, calm, peace)
Lycopodium (expanding into the fullness of who you are)
Oak (grounding, aligning, balancing, unifying)
Silica (moving things through)
Sulphur (spinning out,
Rainbow (self-love)
Thuja (revealing, uncovering, grounding, detoxification)
T-Rex (purification, anti-inflammatory)
Tuberculinum (freedom, expansion, creativity, authenticity)
Vernix (greater feeling of safety, of feeling protected)
All other sacred geometry remedies

Prescribing notes

Potency

1) Please see the chapter on potencies. 30c is mostly what I use and recommend.

2) General Prescribing

As well as being prescribed as a remedy in it's own right, the Golden Spiral can provide a lovely support to other remedies, as they do their work; working alongside those remedies to help the vital force spiral out the dis-ease. The Golden Spiral can
give more energy to existing remedies to do their work.

3) Skin Aggravations

There can be mild skin aggravations with this remedy, as it spirals out dis-ease, which is another reason why lower potencies would be better. These are very rare.

4) Water purification

This remedy can be added to water to help purify it. It's best to leave it overnight. Just one 30c pillule or a drop of medicating potency in a vat of water. It works beautifully with Flower of Life too for water purification.

5) Detoxification

Golden Spiral combines well with Flower of Life, Thuja & Silica 30c to make a detox remedy that has been tested using kinesiology to work with detoxing the COVID vaccines.

This is what I do instead of giving these vaccines in potency, as I didn't resonate with the energy of the vials of these vaccines in potencies. Given one three times a day for 5-7 days then one daily for another 21 days. This can be repeated if needed.

Golden Spiral can also be given as a Saturday remedy when following standard detoxification protocols. I do use standard protocols (Ton Jansen) for all other detoxification.

6) Cancer

This is a remedy that can be given to people receiving allopathic treatment for cancer to support the system in processing the drugs. I give this, along with Flower of Life as part of the relevant Golden Spiral Sarcode for the part of the body that is affected. This combines detoxification with organ support.

I really like giving the Guild Mega Chemo mix 30x (yes, 30x is the correct potency) that is sold by Helios to help clear the effects of any allopathic treatment too, and then a constitutional if it feels appropriate too.

This is a remedy that supports the soul to align with path ahead - if the person is to stay on Earth, this remedy will help the person to align with their next steps ahead, and call in the support that they need. If it is the soul's journey to leave this Earth, this remedy will support them in their next steps.

I have seen a remarkable case of a person with cancer in a family of people who weren't interested in homeopathy, apart from a relative of the person with cancer, who sent Golden Spiral + Flower of Life 30c to every member of the wider family, and asked everyone to take one a day, as a way of clearing any ancestral or family issues that may have contributed to the person getting cancer that did.

This approach has been remarkable to behold.

7) Colds & Flus

Golden Spiral + Flower of Life seems to be great at working with colds and flus that people get stuck with - Flower of Life opens and purifies all the cells and literally enables people to breathe. I have seen it work instantly in some cases, in others alongside other indicated remedies. I myself will take a 50M of the two together in this situation, but most people cannot take such high potencies. 30c every hour for 3 doses will be great for most people.

8) A Final Thought for Gardeners!

It's easy to image that this remedy would be wonderful for gardening, that plants would love this added to the water they are fed.

In fact, in a simple double-blind experiment I conducted, testing different remedies on the growth of sugar snap pea seeds, the Golden Spiral generated the greatest growth of both stems and deep roots. A video of this experiment is available on the home page of my website.

'There are no limits to what this remedy can do'.

Case Studies

Case Study 1

KC is a 42 year old woman, who initially sought homeopathy for pain in her right shoulder and right lumbar area. During the session the levels of trauma that she had been through emerged. Her mother was co-dependent on her, and KC felt like she was the mother not the child in their relationship. She knew who her father was, but this was a closely guarded secret in the family, which meant that she couldn't have an open relationship with him as her father. She was experiencing problems in her marriage. She was struggling with her weight, and with having a routine of self-care in her life. She was challenged in setting healthy boundaries that loved and honoured her needs. She was in burn out from her work in social care and on sick leave when we started working together.

KC had been having homoepathy for 16 months, during which time she had been able to set healthy boundaries with her mother, her back issues had cleared up, and her relationship with her husband had become close once more. She had returned to work.

At the point when Golden Spiral as a remedy had come into existence, KC had started to cycle back into old behaviour patterns. She was struggling with stress at work, and didn't feel in her body. She was wondering what her purpose in life was. She was having a great and positive impact on clients, but the administration and management of her role was too much for her. She started to reflect on how she wanted to build her life around her wants and wishes. For the first time since living in her city, where she had been for 5 years, she wanted to make friends, and realised she hadn't.

In the first month of taking the Golden Spiral, KC had been emotional, doing lots of crying. She felt she was grieving for herself –

seeing the struggle she had been through for years and how she hadn't loved herself. Other grief came up too – suppressed grief of some of her deceased relatives, as well the impact of lockdown.
She was still reflecting on what she wanted to do with her life in terms of her purpose.

In the second month, she experienced feeling more grounded. Her relationship with her husband had never been better. The positive impact she was having on patients seemed to increase, and she described her work as "incredible". She felt really happy, all of life "felt good". She described making choices that were better for her, communicating her needs more clearly, and knowing what she wants. She decided to commit to a course of study in a new profession that would still have her seeing clients, but in a more empowered way, self-employed, without the same demands for admin that tires her. She described that "everything is re-jigging into it's right place, so that I am in the centre of it".

Case Study 2

RC is a 46 year old woman, who initially sought homeopathy for help with overall wellbeing and balance in body and mind. She experienced tangible headaches and migraines, which would make her very anxious about her health. She struggles with being overweight.

RC is a mother to a young child, separated from the father, who barely sees his child.

RC had been living with her parents for 18 months due to being on a low income, which was stressful for her, as her Mum is domineering with early onset Alzheimer's. RC is very close to her Dad. Her and her son had recently moved into their own flat.
RC's brother is seriously mentally unwell, and RC gets anxious worrying about how she'll have to look after him once her mother

and father die.

RC reported really strong cravings for sugar. Home is very important to her, she needs stability, and the instability caused by the end of her relationship and being home with parents had been hard. She can get quite down.

RC was given Golden Spiral 30c alongside remedies to support her hormones, daily for one month.

RC reported that Golden Spiral had "lifted her up out of being down", and that it had also lifted her out of being stuck – she had been feeling really stuck. She consciously reduced her sugar intake and was really disciplined about it, and started a candida detox. RC is a very grounded person, and a people pleaser. She doesn't like to ask for help with anything from anyone, I was really surprised because on 3 occasions during the follow-up session, she made a point of telling me that the Golden Spiral had run out. The last time in fact, at the end of her call, she almost had the fervour of an addict, and made me promise I would send more.

I didn't see her for another 7 months, as she had been doing so well. In that time, she had started studying for a professional qualification that she had dreamed she would do, and her and her child had moved into a more affordable and more permanent home.

Case Study 3

Mother of 3, 49 years old.

CS had been diagnosed with several autoimmune conditions - Lupus, myosotis, Hashimotos, Raynauds. Her husband comes from a different religion, and so she hid her relationship with him for 3 years before telling her family. All accepted him except a beloved grandparent who died shortly after the news. CS blamed herself for the death.

Extreme fatigue. Digestive issues. She was taking methoxetrate, mepacrine, prednisolone, rituximab IVs, plus others, and antidepressants at start of the case. She had been on steroids for 20 years.Regular infections and antibiotics. Fully COVID vaccinated.

Headstrong. Stoic. Doesn't cry.
Also history of issues with eating since child. anorexia. Although in early consults, this wasn't mentioned more than once in passing - her focus was on the fatigue and autoimmunity so the focus went there.

Her vital force did not respond to bowel nosodes, lanthanides, working with sarcodes (bone marrow, blood cells, spleen, liver, mitochondria), detox protocols, grief remedies, Nat Mur, Ignatia, Arsenicum, Nux, Carc, Syph, Thuja.
Then in one session, just as she was about to give up (her husband had said he had a good feeling for her to carry on), she mentioned the anorexia in passing for only the second time.

Re-repping led me to Tarentula hisp. I asked her if she loved music and dancing and whether she just had to dance when music came on. She started to cry about how much she missed dancing, how it's her favourite thing in the world. I thought about her hiding her relationship.

I prescribed Tarentula hisp 200c twice daily with Phos Ac 200c (combined) In the following session, she described having had a breakdown. She made daily trips to the accident and emergency room, begging for tests. She thought she had cancer and was dying. She felt suicidal. She had been writing goodbye letters to her family.

I prescribed Aurum 10M daily for three days then weekly plus Golden

Spiral 1M daily.

In the following session, for first time in years she described feeling better, her energy was better, her muscles were working better, she had started EATING, she had gained weight, had a trial session with a therapist that went well, had talked to doctor about coming off antidepressants who was supporting her wish, she had found her mojo, felt like a different person, and had decided she REFUSED to be ill anymore.

I literally watched her vital force roar back to life. It was really profound to witness.

The Flower of Life

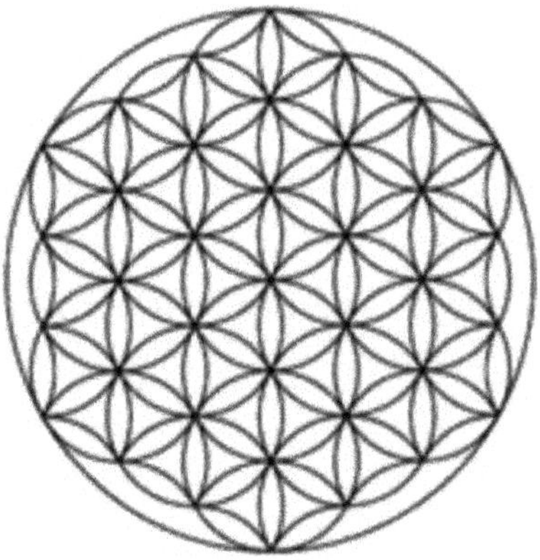

"Embedded in the Flower of Life, just as with the Golden Spiral, is the vibration of love."

This proving took place on 27th November 2023, during the Full Moon in Gemini, which was a Full Moon with the theme of communication, expressing emotions, vulnerability & family. [25]

It was a time of reflecting on the needs of our inner emotional landscape & our inner child(ren), reflecting on patterns that help us & patterns that can sabotage us. The energy of this Full Moon including speaking one's truth to others, and being accountable for ourselves. Neptune was in a supportive trine aspect to Venus in Scorpio, which enables us to relate to one another from a higher aspect; through loving kindness, compassion, open-heartedness & empathy.

11 provers were involved in the first proving of this remedy. 10 of the provers were women, and 1 man was involved. A range of potencies were taken by the provers from 30c to 10M.

The making of this remedy

The remedy was made by triturating up to a 6c using Dr Paul Theriault's teachings, to send the energy of the remedy through the physical, emotional, mental and spiritual layers of consciousness and through into the collective. Higher potencies were then made from there.

---

25 https://www.amybirdartandastrology.com/blog

This remedy was made between the 10th and 29th October 2023.

The Flower of Life

The Flower of Life is a sacred geometry symbol made from "19 intersecting circles (that are actually spheres) spaced evenly from each other that reveal an intricate pattern of overlapping symmetrical flowers".

The number 19 is considered to be significant, particularly according to some scholars of the Quran, following the theory of Dr Rashid Khalifa's, Code 19, which has found the number 19 to be of great significance throughout the Quran. Also:

1. it is a prime number, devisable only by itself and one
2. It is made of the numbers 1 and 9 - new beginnings, and completion; the start and end or the "Alpha and Omega".
3. Number 19 is the numerical value of the word ONE in Arabic gematria.[26]

The Flower of Life is said to promote healing, to protect our energy field, to expand our consciousness, and some believe that the Akashic Records – records and knowledge of all of life – are found in this symbol. The Flower of Life symbolises interconnectedness, unity, oneness, the cycle of life, and the union of divine masculine and feminine energies.

The Flower of Life is our energetic blueprint when we are strong & whole, and it is said to be the blueprint of the universe.

Every single expression of the sacred geometry of our existence can be found within the Flower of Life – it expresses all of the patterns

---

26 https://nassirsabah.com/insights/supplements/the-virgin-mary-and-the-number-19-in-the-quran/

found in our universe. This is the geometry of who we are. For example, it contains within it the Golden Spiral, Vesica Piscis, Tree of Life, Seed of Life, Egg of Life, Fruit of Life, Grid of Life, Torus, Merkabah, the Platonic solids.

How our cells develop when we are conceived directly replicates how the Flower of Life is formed, as this image clearly shows.[27] At the point of conception, we have the circle, which the divides into 2 cells (the Vesica Piscis geometric symbol), from there into 4 cells, then 8 (the Seed of Life), and then to the Flower of Life.

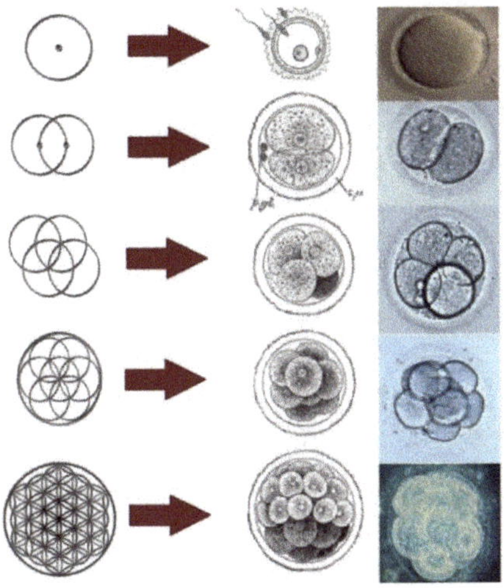

In his remarkable works *The Ancient Secret of the Flower of Life, Volumes 1, 2 & 3, Drunvalo Melchizedek describes in considerable detail the significance of the Flower of Life.*

Drunvalo has travelled the world studying how ancient civilisations understood sacred geometry – from the days of Atlantis, through to the ancient Dogon tribe who can still be found living in Mali in West Africa, to the Ancient Egyptians, who had the Flower of Life symbol depicted in some of their temples, including the temple in Abydos.

27 https://blogs.uoregon.edu/celeah/the-flower-of-life/

The Flower of Life is actually found all around the world including in Ireland, Turkey, England, Israel, Egypt, China, Tibet, and Japan. It is found in the Sikh Golden Temple in Amritsar (India), in a Buddhist Temple in Ajanta (India), in the Louvre and at Ephesus in Greece.

Drunvalo describes how Thoth, the Scribe in Ancient Egypt, had taught Pythagoras about geometry & the nature of reality – including that of the Flower of Life.

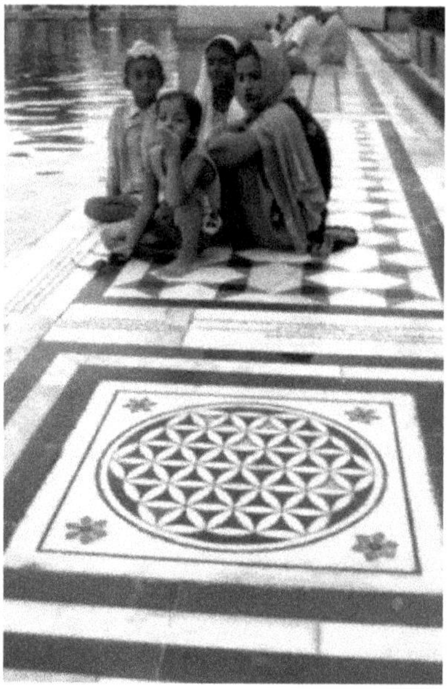

"When Egypt died, it was Thoth who started the next major culture, which was Greece. Our history books say that Pythagoras was the father of Greece and that it was from and through the Pythagorean school that Greece unfolded and from Greece that our present civilisation emerged. Pythagoras says in his own writings that Thoth took him by the hand, led him under the Great Pyramid and taught him all the geometries and the nature of the Reality."

Drunvalo goes on to describe how everything in reality is expressed as a wave – more specifically a sine wave. The sine waves correspond to light and sound – including to the electromagnetic spectrum. The Flower of Life contains all of the mathematics found in the sine wave expression of energy and life.

Golden Spiral in the Flower of Life (an expression of the flow of life, found in every aspect of nature including in human bodies, the spiral of the DNA, in how chakras flow, how the soul enters and leaves the body, plants, how currents in the oceans flow and how planets orbit each other through the solar system)

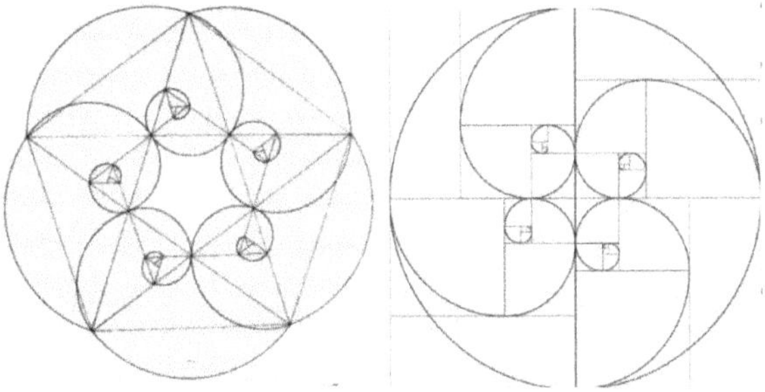

Tree of Life in the Flower of Life (this represents the pathway of our soul to Source / God Each of the circles (Sephirot) corresponds to an important aspect of life that is part of the journey to Source. These include Keter (closest to Source), Binah (understanding), Chochmah (wisdom), Da'at (knowledge - this one can be hidden), Gemurah (strength of boundaries), Chesed (loving & kindness), Tifaret (harmony & beauty), Hod (surrender), Netzach (victory), Yesod (foundation), Malkut (manifestation & sovereignty). The Tree of Life connects us with boundaries as well as with love & also balances the masculine & feminine.

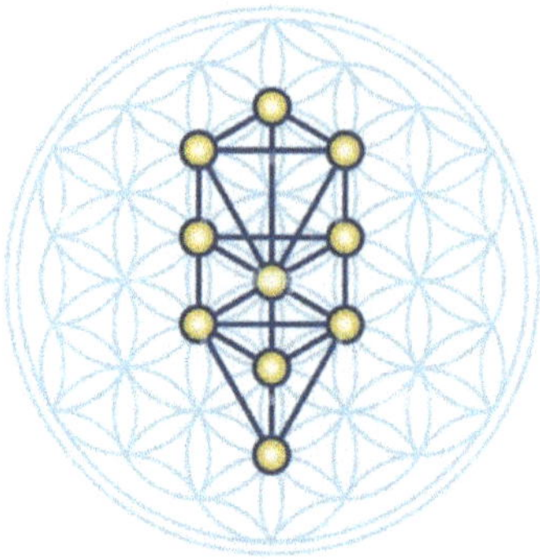

Seed of Life within the Flower of Life (The Seed of Life consists of 7 circles that overlap & represents the 7 days of creation. It is the seed of the Flower of Life. The Seed of Life connects with how life starts from a seed, and then blossoms and grows – just like the universe has done. It also corresponds to exactly how a 3 day old embryo looks - the point at which it becomes a multicellular organism.)

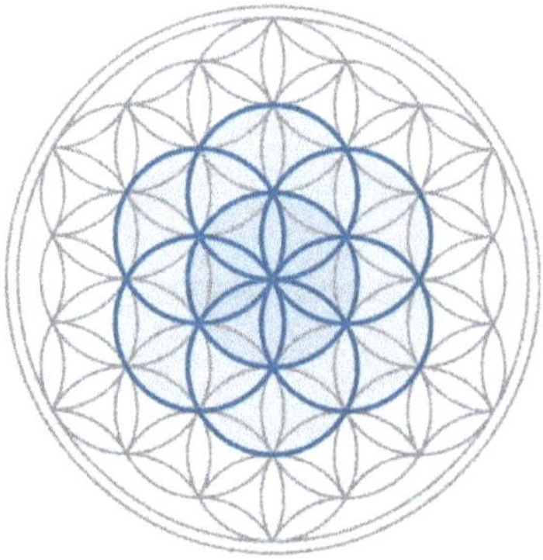

Fruit of Life within the Flower of Life (This is composed of 13 spheres. 13 represents unity & connection through dimensions & worlds. In a chromatic scale of 12 notes, there is a 13 - it's the same note as the first, but another octave higher, representing moving into a higher dimension.

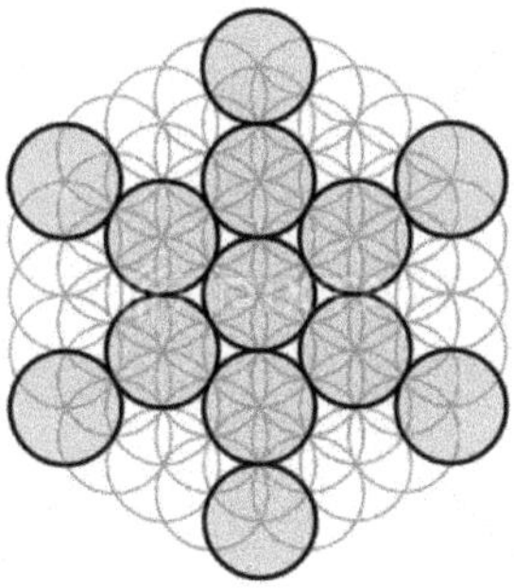

13 is also the number of the Divine Feminine; 13 moons in a calendar year, and so 13 menstrual (lunar) cycles. In Ancient Egypt, 13 represented the joyous afterlife. The Fruit of Life encourages us to move towards our desires & goals; turning our aspirations into a reality, just like the Divine Feminine materialises what is a desire into physical material form in order to become mothers).

Egg of Life within the Flower of Life (The Egg of Life represents the stage of growth of the embryo when it has divided into 4 and then into 8 cells; this is the sacred geometry of the egg of life).

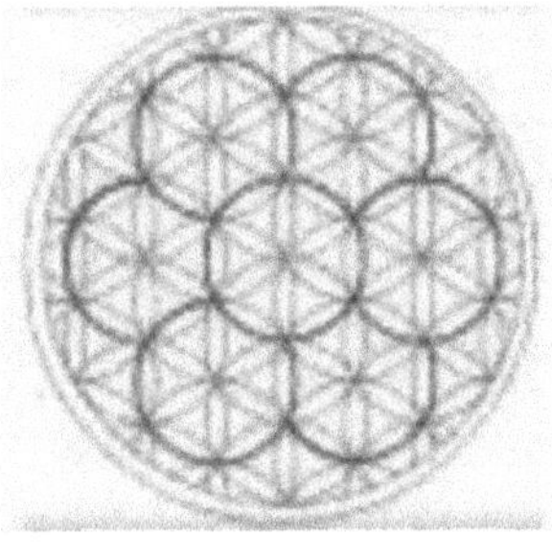

We also see the Platonic solids in the Flower of Life. Named after Ancient Greek philosopher Plato (347 BC), these are the geometric shapes that make up all of life and the universe. They are made of polygons or *polyhedra,* which in Greek means "many faces", where each face, edge and angel between each face is identical. Each one in 2D expands further until we would eventually see a circle form.

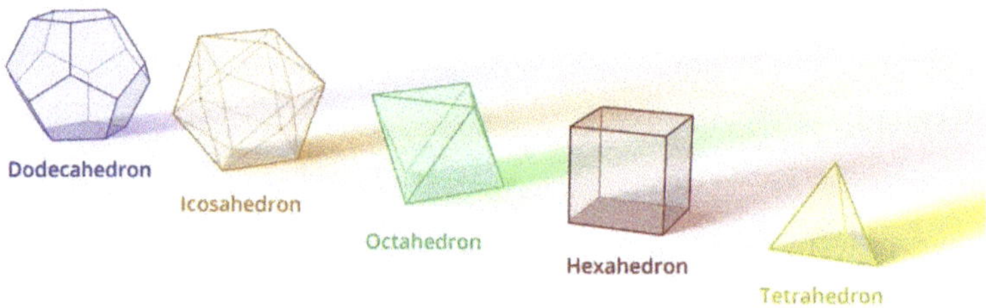

Some say that Pythagoras had described these 200 years earlier, calling them the "Perfect Solids".[28]

The Platonic solids are 3D polygons or polyhedra, and because of the mathematics of making these 2D shapes 3D, only 5 Platonic solids can exist:

Tetrahedron (4 faces of triangles; a pyramid or tetrahedron)
Hexahedron (6 faces of squares; a cube)
Octahedron (8 faces of triangles; a diamond)
Dodecahedron (12 faces of pentagons)
Icosahedron (20 faces of triangles).

Metatron's Cube is a symbol found in the Flower of Life, built from the Fruit of Life, that also contains all of the Platonic Solids. A beautiful video depicting how this happens can be found using the link in this

28 https://www.sacredgeometryshop.com/sacred-geometry/the-secrets-of-the-platonic-solids/

footnote.[29]

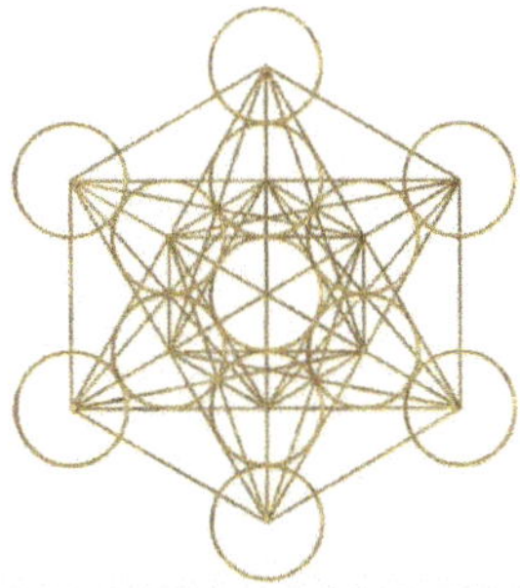

Merkabah (Made of two tetrahedrons that intersect & rotate in opposite directions, which creates an energy field known as the light body (Torus) once spinning. It is said that connecting with one's Merkabah can provide powerful protection, enabling us to access higher consciousness. In Chassidic Judaism, the Merkabah aligns us with all the aspects of life, the natural world, and the Earth too.)

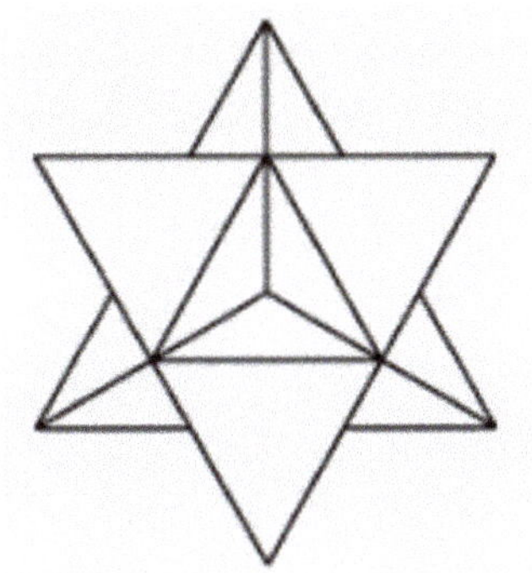

Torus (The Torus is a type of vortex & is what our aura, or energetic - electromagnetic - field looks like. When our aura isn't strong, we can feel more sensitive, or more emotionally challenged. Sometimes energies can flow in a way that generates more negative emotions. When the Toroidal field is out of balance, toxic emotions, narcissism, sociopathy & psychopathy can set in.

---

29 https://www.sacredgeometryshop.com/sacred-geometry/the-secrets-of-the-platonic-solids/

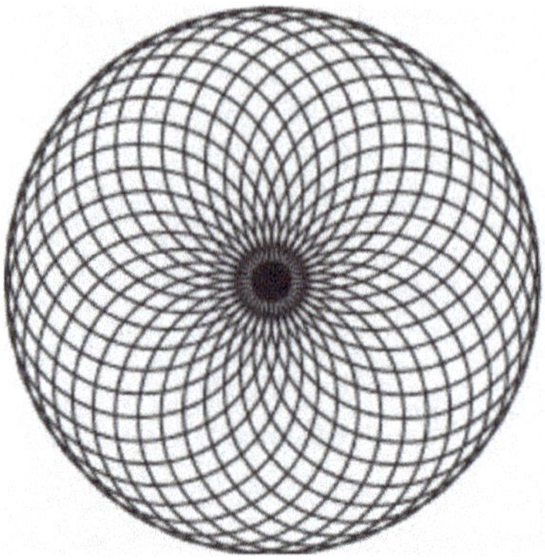

We find the Flower of Life in the Vitruvian Man by Leonardo da Vinci around 1490. This beautiful Vitruvian Woman has been drawn by homeopath Joanne Camlin whilst connecting with the Flower of Life. Joanne has kindly given her permission for us to share her artwork in this proving.

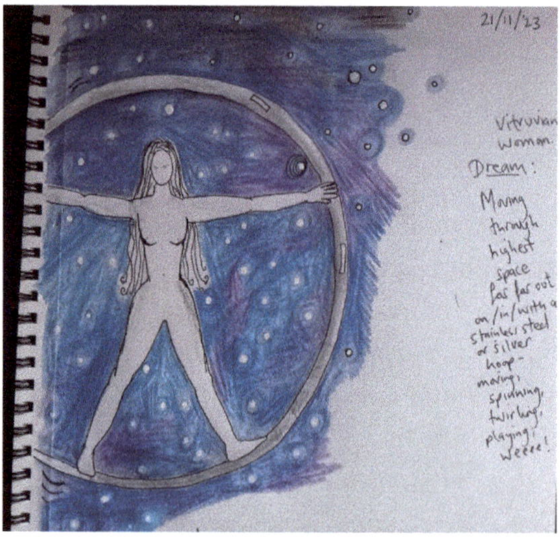
21/11/23
Vitruvian Woman.
Dream:
Moving through highest space far far out on/in/with a stainless steel or silver hoop - moving, spinning, twirling, playing! Weeee!

Flower of Life Homeopathic Remedy™

Key Themes

Expansion
Breathing
Light
Activations, Higher consciousness & awakening
Multidimensional
War trauma
Grief & sadness
Anger
Anxiety
Self-consciousness, worth & value
Clears darkness
Overview of life; brings ease & spaciousness
Peace
Truth
Gratitude
Energising
Abundance
Heals relationships, connects with communities
Protection
Blood
Life

Key Themes

Expansion

This remedy brings expansion. Several provers experienced huge expansions in the heart area. Where there is anxiety in the heart that can cause difficulties with a person allowing their heart to be open & expansive, this remedy clears the anxiety so that the heart can expand.

Breathing

The expansion was also experienced in the lungs with several provers noting the ability to breathe and expand the lungs more easily thank usual. This is a remedy that can clear what is in the lungs.

Light

This is a remedy that connects us with light. It literally brings a lighter vibration with it; it shines a light in the darkness, like the remedy Ayahuasca.

Activations, Higher Consciousness & Awakening

The Flower of Life brings activations at a cellular level, and throughout the mind, body & soul. This includes the DNA, pineal gland & brain activations.

As one prover said: This is part of the DNA: [I am] assimilating information, making it part of me, making it close, amalgamating, merging, integrating, assimilating, consuming."

There was a reminder with the Flower of Life of the activations that the Eye of Horus bring.

The Eye of Horus according to the Ancient Egyptians represents powerful activations in the brain, body and soul.

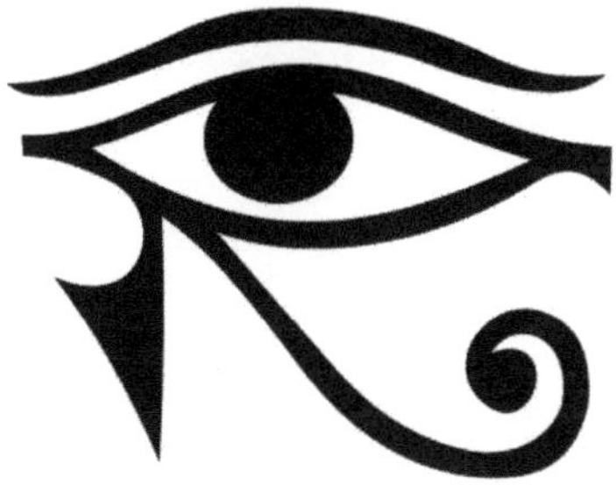

The eyebrow signifies the *corpus callosum*, the bridge that connects the right and left hemispheres of the brain. This aspect of the Eye of Horus unites the left and right halves of the brain; uniting logic and intuition, the head and the heart, knowing and sensing.
This is said to connect us with wisdom.

The outline of the eye represents the *thalamus,* which regulates consciousness.

The pupil represents the *pineal gland,* which connects with intuition and higher consciousness.

The downward line represents the *hypothalamus*, which secretes hormones. Hormones are physical chemical messengers in the body, but are also said spiritually to also be messengers with the Cosmos. Some say that this is why menstruating women can have greater intuitive abilities, as our hormones can help us to feel a greater emotional and spiritual connection. This is why taking synthetic hormones that suppress our endocrine system, can also our intuition and spiritual connections.

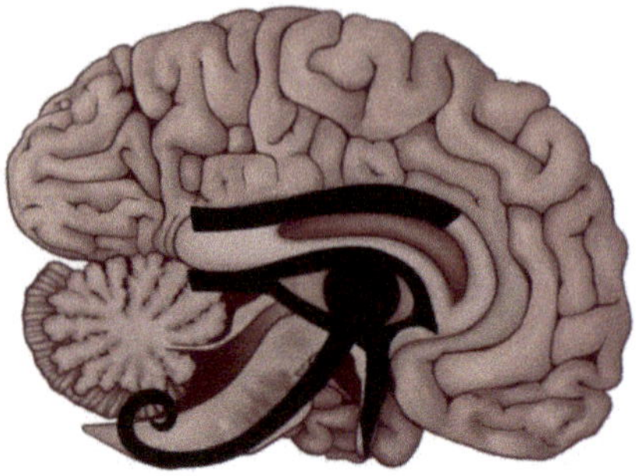

The senses are also represented in the Eye of Horus; taste, hearing, seeing, touch & smell. This is how we receive information energetically & metaphysically.[30]

It is no coincidence that we are often shown an eye enclosed in a triangle – this represents the shutting down or control of all of these aspects of our consciousness.

The Flower of Life activates & reawakens our consciousness, transcending any limitations that we may have encountered.

Multidimensional

The Flower of Life is a remedy that transcends time & space. Several provers experienced connecting with other dimensions, including two provers who connected with angels.

Within the Flower of Life, we have Metatron's Cube, named after Archangel Metatron. Archangel Metatron is said to have been one of only 2 angels that have ever lived on Earth; that he and Archangel

30 https://www.ncbi.nlm.nih.gov/pmc/articles/PMC6649877/

Sandalphon were the twin brothers Enoch and Elijah, the sons of Abraham.
The Keys of Enoch[31] is a book with the nickname "Metatron's Book", for it describes in much detail the metaphysics of the divine electron, energy, sound, language, our energy fields, and life on Earth and in the cosmos.

It makes sense that angels would therefore – also as an expression of love, and the bringing of healing – are an important part of this remedy.

War trauma

It was during the trituration of this remedy (when trituating 1c) that Israel started bombing Palestine in October 2023. Several provers connected deeply with the situation in Israel & Palestine.

One prover was reminded of her grandfather was in a work camp during WW2.

This remedy brings peace where there has been war. This is may be a useful remedy to add to water and the land and to take when meditating on peace. This remedy may also bring healing to the physical effects of war. One prover, for example, experienced stopped up ears: "as though after a bomb has gone off and then you can't hear anything".

Trauma affects the integrity of the energy field. The wonderful late Dr Masuro Emoto has proved what happens when you place water over the words love and then hate.

The energy of hate causes the perfect geometry of water to collapse into non-geomtric blobs. The energy of love supports the

31 8 J. J. Hurtak (1977) *The Keys of Enoch* The Academy for Future Science

integrity of amazing geometry in the water – and can turn polluted or hate-filled water back into perfectly geometric "love water".

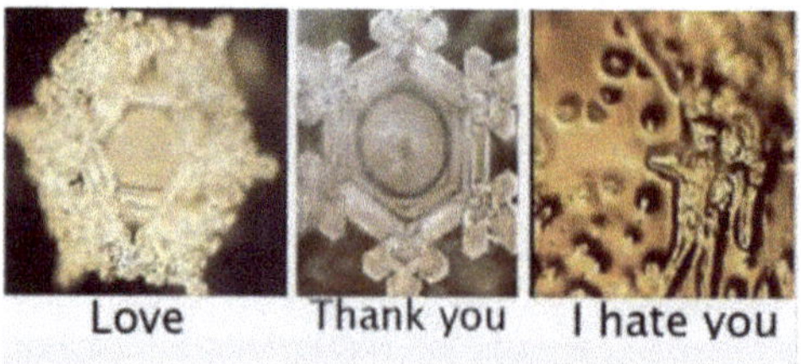

In the *Trauma, beyond the Patriarchy and Remedies for a New Earth* course, I describe what I have come to understand from channellings I have received about how trauma affects our energy field.

If this is what we know happens to water, then this is definitely what happens to the geometry of our energy field – our blueprint, the Flower of Life (and the Golden Spiral, Fruit of Life, Egg of Life, Tree of Life, Merkabah, Torus, the Platonic Solids and all of the geometry with which our life is expressed) loses it's geometric structure.

This is what trauma does to our field.

This is one of the remedies – along with the other geometric remedies that we now have – that reverses the damage that trauma does to the integrity of our energy field' our sacred geometry; our blueprint.

Grief & sadness

This remedy bring considerable heart healing, and one prover compared it with Thymus Gland and Green.

Anger

We found that Flower of Life brought healing to two types of anger: the kind of anger we see with grief (like ignatia), and also the kind of anger that is about injustice (like causticum).

There was a need to speak about the truth, and to speak up about the issues that matter.

Anxiety

Anxiety is a key theme with the Flower of Life. Several provers described feeling anxious, struggling to breathe with it, feeling the anxiety in their heart. As one prover said:

"I was overwhelmed with anxiety.......I had to take an Aconite 10M to get rid of it......it was like I could see spinning ball, a sphere in front of me, it was resting on my chest, and I could feel [other people's] feet spinning it and pressing it down. You know when you're really upset and you try to take a breath in and you almost judder? And I could really exhale long, and slow and it was like "how the fuck can I exhale like this when I can't even take an in-breath? So anxiety with no inhalation but a long exhalation, and this sphere on the chest. It felt like all of humanity was pushing that ball on my chest".

This remedy brings peace to anxiety.

Self-consciousness, worth & value

The Flower of Life reminds us of our worth and value. One prover had a school reunion around the time of the proving. She had gone to a private school where the women had either a) married into wealth after school and never worked or b) had often not just become doctors, lawyer, politicians or film directors.....they had risen to the top of their profession.

The prover described it like this: "I loved my school, but I was a fish out of water. I came from a working class background, and going to this reunion I realised that the women all just grew up knowing their own worth – that they are literally *treasure.* This remedy has helped me realise that I am treasure too – not from a place of ego, but from a place of acceptance of my worth. It's been really liberating."
This is another way in which this remedy connects us with the perfection of who we are, reminding us that we don't need cosmetic surgery and interventions.

During the proving it was felt that this could be a remedy for those who have had, or are thinking of having, Botox, lip augmentation or cosmetic work that alters their natural beauty.

Clears darkness

We have already discussed this remedy in terms of war trauma; some of the most syphilitic and dark energies that we can be clearing as homeopaths.

Also, where there is darkness due to the energy field not being intact, or being compromised, the Flower of Life helps to remedy this.

Overview of life; brings ease & spaciousness

The Flower of Life brings us an overview of life, like the bird remedies do. It reminds us of the smallness of us & our lives on this one planet travelling through the cosmos filled with billions of stars & planets.

Birds were a theme with this remedy – especially the energy of parrot / macaw. 3 provers mentioned parrots!

I noticed how many things in my life were happening with grace and ease. I have always used a marble pestle and mortar when triturating, and came across a porcelain one in a shop that I bought to and when I used it to make the remedy, I thought "wow! It's sooooo much lighter and easier to use! Where have I been? It's almost effortless!"

People who could help with the next level of work stepped in, bringing more support, and making life easier. This brought more spaciousness in life.

With the energy field more intact, we are less likely to feel like we are wading through treacle. One of the key themes of this remedy is relationships; it made it easier to bring helpers in, and gently can clear more draining connections. This would be a natural consequence of a more integral energy field.

Peace

One prover saw a white dove when thinking about her grandfather who was in a work camp in WW2, and instinctively felt this remedy brings peace where there has been war trauma.

The peace was very much felt in the body; clearing anxiety in the heart, so that there was more peace in the heart, and also in the lungs, making it easier to breathe.

Truth

Truth revealed so that healing can occur. The remedy does this gently. With Petrified Sequoia we saw truths being revealed in strong ways at times, whereas the Flower of Life ensures that truths emerge in ways in which the person feels supported and held, even if energetically.

Another aspect of truth the Flower of Life connects with is the truth of who we are. It reminds us of our nature; our beauty; our perfection. The Flower of Life itself is perfect. We are are an expression of that perfection.

During the proving it was felt that this could be a remedy for those who have had, or are thinking of having, Botox, lip augmentation or cosmetic work that alters their natural beauty.

One prover wrote "this is who I am" in relation to this remedy. Two provers connected with the work of Robert F Kennedy Jr, and one with Julian Assange. This is a remedy very much for truth seekers and truth speakers, and supports speaking truth.

One prover was warned not to talk about vaccine damage when giving a talk, which generated a lot of nervousness for her. The prover worked through the nervousness and then chose to speak her truth. She described it as follows.

We are in a new era of homeopathy. We need to break out of the box. What we're doing now is not walking. There are too many sick kids". I spoke my truth with a lot of anger inside, because I'm upset about what's happening to the kids. The talk was great, it was super well received. I did talk about vaccine damage. I didn't let what they told me to rule".

I lost my voice after the talk. Afterwards in a conversation with another homeopath, I realised that I needed the Macaw remedy – which is all about speaking your truth! I keep wanting to take this remedy – I feel like it will bring my strength back to me in this way."

Another prover had had a similar experience, of speaking to a private group online about vaccines, having not spoken about them since Covid online, and found that her video was taken down from You Tube. She said "I just couldn't stay silent anymore."

Despite there being anger in the remedy, the actual sharing of truth comes from a place of presence rather than anger. This is reflective of a more healed energy field.

Gratitude

This remedy brings gratitude for life, and for the smallest things. Several provers described feeling gratitude in different ways; for old friendships even though they no longer existed, for each other, for the beauty of nature, beautiful sunsets, our homes, the people in our lives now.

This remedy heightens our awareness of the wonderful gifts and blessings in our lives; we feel more connected to them through the expansion that we feel.

Energising

This remedy reawakens our natural energetic integrity and strength, and brings an expansiveness to our heart, lungs, brain, consciousness and all of our chakras.

It follows that this remedy is energising; it stimulates the vital force, and is useful where the vital force is depleted.

Abundance

As one prover described, "this a remedy that brings magic and abundance". A more aligned and healed energy field is able to receive energies that sustain and nourish – and this includes relationships that do so, and abundance.

Heals relationships, connects with communities

The Flower of Life connects, brings support, soul connections, being taken care of, clears those where there isn't resonance or respect. As one prover said "This is a remedy that transcends the patriarchy and shows new ways to live and be that are about community and connection – it brings freedom & release".

Protects the body, mind and soul

The protective aspects of this remedy – and it's use in potentially difficult world situations - were beautifully illustrated by a dream that one of the provers had.

The dream was of Russia invading the country the prover lives in. She said "Planes are coming. I live next to the President's castle, on the top floor, so I would be one of first hit. An announcement was made on my phone "you have half an hour to move yourself into rehabilitation centre" which is 20 minutes away from where I live. In every building in [my city], you can go into the basement where there is a bomb shelter, so I was like "what the fuck?". I wondered where my adult children were – are we going together? There was an announcement "the Government is taking over your phone" and then there was nothing. My daughter was still holding the phone, and where we were looking at it, it was showing a bird's eye perspective of the different centres you could move into and it said "this one is full". "This one is full." "This one is full.". There was an awareness that when you take the car, they will take the car away from you because the Government needs it. I was like "what am I going to do?" Then I went into this area in [my city] where I used to live, where there is a lot of space. These people were like "we are not going anywhere, we are staying at home. Just come with us. Don't go to that crazy place. There were people playing saxophone. I went to my office, choosing my machine and remedies to take with me because I know I am the medicine woman, knowing what to take with me."

It was really interesting that during the writing of this proving, a friend and colleague had told me about a new film on Netflix starring Julia Roberts called *Leave the World Behind.* There was one point during the writing up of this proving that I just HAD to watch it; as though I couldn't continue the write up without watching it.

It's a film that depicts what happens during a fictional cyber attack to two families. It has resonance with what the prover had described in her dream.

It reminded me of what we found during the proving of the Survivor Tree remedy. It is made from the one tree found still growing in Ground Zero after 9/11 happened, and is a remedy gifted to us thanks to homeopaths Hilery Dorrian and Maggie Dixon. One of the key themes of the remedy is it's invincibility. That particular species of tree – a type of very small ornamental pear tree, *Pyrus calleryana* – is naturally resistant to fire and pests. During the proving, we connected with it literally having a force field to protect itself with.

It feels relevant to share a part of the that proving here, to explain a feature of Flower of Life.

"There is a theory about what happened in 9/11 proposed by physicist Dr Judy Wood who wrote Where Did The Towers Go? Evidence of Directed Free Energy Technology on *9/11.*[32] She has lectured extensively and can be found on YouTube discussing the question of why there wasn't a gargantuan pile up of rubble after the Twin Towers collapsed. There was, however, a lot of *dust.* She

32 Dr Judy Wood (2010) Where Did The Towers Go? Evidence of Directed Free Energy Technology on 9/11

plays the video footage slowly to demonstrate her theory that a Direct Energy Weapon (DEW) was used at the time the planes hit; which caused vaporisation and dust, rather than a lot of rubble, as would be expected.

We are moving into a time when there are increasing conversations about radiation in many different forms; from mobile phone radiation to 5G towers to the use of bluetooth and microwave technology and very recently DEWs; some claim that DEWs are the cause of many of the forest fires we are seeing.

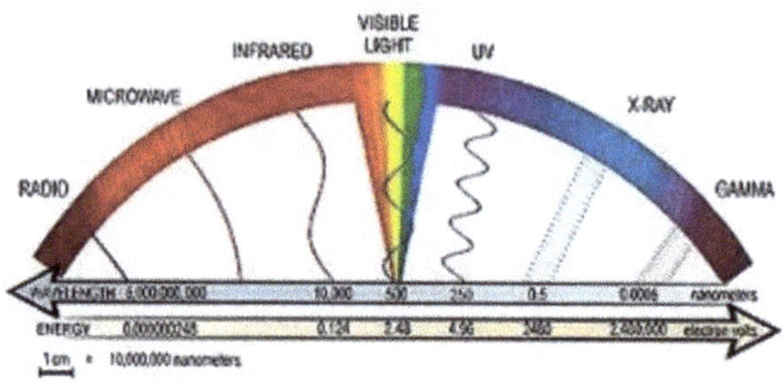

In the provings, we don't take a view on these perspectives, however it may be that nature – and this remedy – is showing us that it is possible to survive and then even thrive no matter the cause of any devastation; even if it could be energy-related.[33]

In the *Leave the World Behind* film, there is a depiction of a potential physical response to DEWs, which begin with a very loud sound and intense pressure in the head followed by neurological and physical symptoms – and reference to an event during 2017 in Cuba where direct microwave energy were actually used.

.

A further conversation with my colleague and friend explored how people's dreams can be accessed, and how people are increasingly

33 https://www.nbcnews.com/news/all/havana-syndrome-likely-caused-microwave-energy-government-study-finds-n1250094

noticing marketing is directed not just according to web searches, or even conversations between friends that the phone may have picked up on, but also simply based on *thoughts* that they are having that they may not have shared with anyone, or google searched.
The Flower of Life remedy reminds of our very blueprint; the geometry of our bodies, minds, and souls. Taking this remedy can act as a protective remedy where this may be needed. The Flower of Life strengthens it from being open to negative influences; supporting the integrity of our being and ensuring that we remain whole and strong.

It may be that a triad combination of Survivor Tree (force field) with Flower of Life (the very structure of what we are) with Mastic Gum (the repair remedy) may be useful in cases such as these.

Blood

A key theme with the Flower of Life is blood. Blood is life within our bodies, carrying the very oxygen we breathe. This remedy can be considered for women working with their fertility. We found that it may help where there is amenorrhoea or dysmenorrhoea.

One prover in particular found that her period was exceptionally and uncharacteristically heavy during her period.

Activates the spine

This remedy is an activator. The spine – bones and teeth – are made of a crystalline structure. Flower of Life reminds and activates the spine as to it's natural state.

Trauma is recorded in the fascia, spine and DNA, and this remedy helps shift that out, bringing greater alignment in the spine. This can bring clearer connections with higher consciousness and the wisdom within it.

Life

The Flower of Life remedy is about life itself. How do we live it? Who are we in it? Who do we welcome in it? How can we at peace with ourselves, in our families and communties? How do we express the greatest version of ourselves? How do we live with the highest consciousness possible?

Also the Flower of Life is an expression of all of LIFE. It connects us with nature, animals, the natural world; seas, oceans, mountains, forests, the sun, the planets. Mama Gaia and our beautiful planet.

Mental & Emotional Symptoms

Anxiety
Scattered thoughts
Difficulties focusing
Restlessness
Wanting to do a million things at the same timeline
Finding the balance between working and living, knowing when to rest
Expansiveness

Physical Particular Symptoms

Head

Throbbing in right temple
Boring pain in the right occiput

Tingling at the back of the head

Eyes

Watery eyes – lachrymation

Ears

Tinnitus in right ear
Clogged
Damage to ears due to war trauma including loss of hearing
Stitching pain in left ear

Nose

Hair growth out of nostril
Pressure in sinuses
Aching of bones in the side of the nose
Thick coryza – clear colour (right nostril)
Lots of sneezing
Itching of the nose (right nostril)

Mouth & Teeth

Tightness in jaw
Clenching of jaw
Teeth grinding
Tingling or numbness in cheeks & jaws
Twitching sensations in right corner of lips
Cold sores / herpes
Mouth ulcer
Furry tongue

Face

Swollen face, red & puffy (allergic reactions)

Throat

Dry
Itchy, scratchy
Raw

Lungs & breathing

Expansiveness – can take in more oxygen
Steady breathing
Asthma
Can be a support to those on a ventilator
Cough – as though clearing dust or dirt that has been breathed in
A clearing cough
Tickly cough
Sleep apnoea
COPD

Heart

Brings expansion to heart
Relaxed, easeful
Anxiety in the heart
Atherosclerosis / Arteriosclerosis
Aneurysm

Stomach

Hungry
Digestion
Candida

Nausea
Morning sickness
SIBO
Parasite imbalance

Kidneys, Bladder, Urination

Increased urination
Proteinuria

Liver

Decongestant for liver
Fibrosis of the liver
Fatty Liver Disease
Gallstones

Reproductive systems

Fertility
Amenorrhoea
Dysmenorrhea
Miscarriage
Enlarged left breast
Morning sickness

Back & Limbs

Aching behind shoulder blades
General aches & pains
Pain in upper spine, between shoulders
Pain in left rib
Oedema

Skin

Excessive sweat
Cold, clammy skin
Fungal infections

Physical General Symptoms

Body Temperature

Cold, chilly
Hot flushes or heat followed by chill
Changing temperatures (mercury)
Shivers

Food & Thirst

Excessive / intense hunger
Thirsty
Desire for cool, clean water
Desire for high vibration, organic, clean foods (this remedy helps people make those
choices)

Dreams

Past relationships
Wars
What matters in life

Sleep

Brings feelings of relaxation, so promotes sleep

Bodily fluids

Congestion of lymph
Poor circulation
Water retention

Energy

Tiredness
Low energy & low vital force
Exhaustion

Clinical

Cancer - all cancers
Herpes
Viral loads
Anaphylaxis
Allergies
Covid clearing remedy
Colds that are difficult to clear
Twitches in different places within the body
Vertigo, very dizzy
Vertigo with nausea
Fungal infection
COPD
Atherosclerosis / Arteriosclerosis
Aneurysm

Spiritual

Flower of Life brings expansion in all ways spiritually, and with all of the chakras. As one prover said "it brings a sparkle to all of the chakras".

Chakras

Crown

More easily able to connect with higher wisdom. Feeling of connection to a higher consciousness.

Third Eye

Stronger intuition, more easily able to experience energy through the intuitive senses.

Throat

Difficulties speaking one's truth. There may be a lot of anger and rage that may be unexpressed, so this chakra may be blocked. Flower of Life can help with speaking truth from a place of presence.

Higher Heart (Thymus Chakra)

This chakra is the point of connection and disconnection physically (with our health, particularly our immunity), and through time with ourselves in all lifetimes. Flower of Life is a multidimensional remedy that calls in an alignment with all parts of ourselves, through time and space

Heart

Flower of Life brings a huge sense of expansion to the heart, and with it peace and gratitude.

Solar plexus

This remedy brings a feeling of being really centred, and aligned with our truth. We know what feels right based on our gut feeling – It's our solar plexus that tells us what resonates and what doesn't resonate - what feels right and what doesn't' feel right, we feel it right there.

Sacral

Where there are energy leaks in relationships, this remedy helps to seal these off, so that energy is no longer being drained in the same way, and the person can feel more whole. This remedy brings healing to past relationships, whether the person gets in contact or not, so that there is peace and a release from the past.

Root

This remedy brings greater expansion & grounding at the Root Chakra, particularly where there has been a scatteredness.

Remedy affinities

Ignatia
Rainbow
Causticum
Thymus Gland
Green
Bird remedies (especially Macaw / Parrot)
Silver Birch
Buddleia

Petrified Sequoia
Syphilinum
Ayahuasca
9/11 Survivor Tree
Aconite

Prescribing notes

1) It may be that a triad combination of Survivor Tree (force field) with Flower of Life (the very structure of what we are) with Mastic Gum (the repair remedy) may be useful in cases such as these.
30c, 200c or 1M up to three times a day as a preventative. 10M or 50M three times a day during times of intensity if the vital force can take it.

2) All of the potencies are useful potencies from 30c up.

3) It combines beautifully with a breathing combination that I use as a therapeutic for those with asthma or other breathing difficulties. Carbo veg, oxygenium, coca & flower of life 1M, to be taken as needed.

4) I use Flower of Life together with Golden Spiral at the first sign of a cold or flu symptoms, either 30c every hour for 3 doses, and then repeat as needed. So far, I have seen it work every single time I have used it with myself or others to clear the vibration and restore vitality.

5) Cancer

This is a remedy that can be given to people receiving allopathic treatment for cancer to support the system in processing the drugs. I give this, along with Flower of Life as part of the relevant Golden Spiral Sarcode for the part of the body that is affected. This combines detoxification with organ support.

I really like giving the Guild Mega Chemo mix 30x (yes, 30x is the correct potency) that is sold by Helios to help clear the effects of any allopathic treatment too, and then a constitutional if it feels appropriate too.

This is a remedy that supports the soul to align with path ahead - if the person is to stay on Earth, this remedy will help the person to align with their next steps ahead, and call in the support that they need. If it is the soul's journey to leave this Earth, this remedy will support them in their next steps.

I have seen a remarkable case of a person with cancer in a family of people who weren't interested in homeopathy, apart from a relative of the person with cancer, who sent Golden Spiral + Flower of Life 30c to every member of the wider family, and asked everyone to take one a day, as a way of clearing any ancestral or family issues that may have contributed to the person getting cancer that did. This approach has been remarkable to behold.

A final note - the Flower of Life as a geometric sarcode of the cell and the energy field

I feel that the Golden Spiral is the geometric sarcode of the DNA and the Flower of Life is the geometric sarcode of the cell, and of the energy field. This is how I work with them, and prescribe them.

Vesica Piscis

14 August 2025
Lilla
Watarrka Land
Northern Territory
Australia

7 provers were involved in the proving of this remedy. All provers were women.

The making of this remedy

The remedy was made by intuitively triturating up to a 12c using Kim Kalina and Dr Paul Theriault's teachings on the levels of trituration, sending the energy of the remedy through the physical, emotional, mental and spiritual layers of consciousness, through into the collective and the planet. Higher potencies were then made from there.

The essence of Vesica Piscis that was then triturated to make the remedy and the remedy itself were made by a Blood Wood Tree. This is a type of Eucalyptus - it is a resilient tree and can regrow easily. The resin it sheds is called Blood Resin and is known for its gluing properties - sticking things together, which is very fitting of what Vesica Piscis represents!

Vesica Piscis

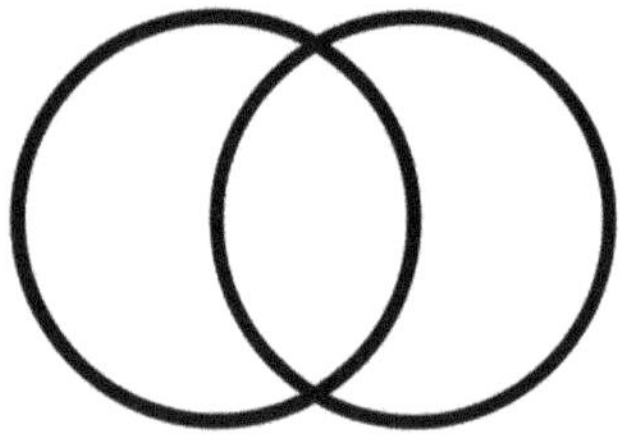

The Vesica Piscis is a shape made of two overlapping circles where each has the same radius, and the centre of each circle lies on thecircumference of the other.

Circles represent the infinite; the one. What we have with the Vesica Piscis is "two overlapping infinite infinites".[34]

"Vesica Piscis" literally means "fish bladder" In the early days of Christianity, Christians often used the fish symbol as a way to identify each other discreetly when they had to lie in greater secret. The shape of the Vesica Piscis resembles the outline of a fish, especially when viewed horizontally. Because of this, the symbol became associated with the sacred fish emblem of Christ. The Vesica Piscis is for this reason an important symbol in Christianity.

The two circles symbolise complementary aspects coming together - masculine and feminine, spirit and matter, self and other, heaven and earth. The overlapping space - the almond-shaped centre - is understood to be the threshold between worlds, the space where opposites meet to generate something new. Many traditions see this central area as a symbol of birth, genesis, and divine manifestation, or materialisation which is why it appears in early Christian art as the *mandorla* surrounding Christ or the Virgin Mary.

As Cassie Uhl says: "If we recognize the circle on its own as Source Energy (God or Goddess, whichever you prefer), the Vesica Piscis represents creation or the "womb of The Universe." Think of a single circle as a Source of Energy, adding a second circle represents the spark of creation when the universe is born. This idea is enforced by

34 https://eyeofheaven.medium.com/the-soul-and-sacred-geometry-the-spiritual-meaning-of-two-circles-the-vesica-piscis-e8887d5254a5

its similarities to the shape of the vagina, the starting place of birth on a human level. It is enforced again by the fact that it is the starting place of most sacred geometry.[35]

For the Pythagoreans, it was a gateway to metaphysical knowledge, a diagram that encoded the hidden harmonies of the cosmos. [36] The proportions embedded within the Vesica Piscis are considered to be foundational. The ratio of its width to its height gives rise to core mathematical constants and geometric constructions, including the square root of 3 and the basis for equilateral triangles (which form the octahedron and tetrahedron Platonic Solids), hexagons (which form the dodecahedron Platonic solid), and the Flower of Life.

The Vesica Piscis also represents the meeting point; a relationship where two separate aspects become connected. It is a reminder that creation emerges through connection.

Vesica Piscis Homeopathic Remedy™

Key Themes

Separation, Division & Connection
Lost Generations
Technology, Connection & Disconnection
Bullying
Shame
Restoration
Grief and Loss
Homesickness
Mediation

---

35 https://www.cassieuhl.com/blog/the-birthplace-of-sacred-geometry-what-is-the-vesica-piscis
36 Stephen Skinner (2009) *Sacred Geometry: Deciphering the Code* Union Square & Co

Loneliness - welcomes a relationship
Grandmothers & Amma
Staying true to self
Re-balancing Masculine and Feminine
Success, harmony & balance
Simplicity
Clarity
Time
Post Natal Depression, Mother & Child Bonding, Issues affecting women & parents
Vision

Separation, Division & Connection

The themes of separation, division and separation were experienced in several ways, including:

- in people being separated from their culture
- the separating of Indigenous children from their parents by settlers (in Australia, but also around the world), and also
- parents and children being separated
- People feeling separated from partners (either real partners, or missing having a partner) - this is a separate keynote.

One prover became really upset at not being able to connect with her children using her phone. The prover stated "At Lilia, i was not getting a phone service or the internet - it felt completely quiet there and remote. I went to my tent to lie down because I felt sort of 'off'. Lying in bed I could feel a panic coming, it felt a little like claustrophobia, I could feel that my children were across the Earth the other side of the globe; they felt far away, and I could not reach them. I took Aconite 200c because I could tell I felt panicky; it felt an unfathomable distance; so quiet there, so remote, I meditated and used my tuning fork to calm myself down. I felt a sense of fear, then I got up and went to join the others. As I started to speak of what I was feeling I started to cry, it felt overwhelming, crushing. Then I cried and [one of the provers] hugged me, and said "I felt that too, I took the bowl and triturated, then I felt better". As I sat with it more, I noticed that I felt like something had been ripped from me; literally like tentacles or a sucubus was taken and I realised it was the cords of the cell phone, some sort of attachment; a cord that made me feel 'connected' to them; it felt like psychic surgery. I saw the aboriginal graph of the family. It says "you are never alone", and shows family, country, land; where you are. With this, you are never alone. That day we had seen the birthing cave, the teaching cave, the sacred water, and I knew I was to learn a new way to feel connected to them - a healthier way, the true way, to know 'I am always connected to them wherever they are; like a cord cutting; a ritual ; to set me and them free; to build our true feeling of connection, our deeper love that is beyond 'worry' and tracking them at every moment, or being able to hear from them whenever I want to. That has replaced or integrated itself into love now. We feel this is love, and I knew I needed to feel liberated; whole within myself and yet connected to them, to the land, our land , our home; that 'I am home wherever I go and so are they."

There was a conversation between this prover and another prover, where the other prover talked about how we can always feel what is happening with our children, even if they are very far away. We *know* deep down if something is wrong.

The prover who was missing her childrenl never got mobile phone service the entire time we were on the land at Lilla where we were staying - and yet thanks to this remedy and the conversations that unfolded from it, she felt "lighter and free".

There was also an awareness that we are returning to young people living with their parents and families more - going back to tribal living structures. This is in part a consequence of global economic pressures on lower and middle income families.

As one prover said: "Covid made it easier to admit that we don't have the money we need to live. People lost their incomes overnight, and it was an accepted consequence. We lost a layer of shame around not having money that we need to live. This was a (positive) unintended consequence of Covid. In addition to this young people don't have access to opportunities to live independently financially as easily, so there isn't the pressure, expectation or shame associated with living at home with parents that there used to be. We are returning to the tribal village ways of living within family systems, and as long as these are supportive and not abusive, this may be positive for everyone, because there is easier connection with support, love, help and it overcomes loneliness."

There was an awareness in the collective of some political issues as well, and the separation that had been generated by this, and the coming together that might be possible to transcend the political challenges.

One prover also talked about the schisms in Christianity, particularly around there having been female disciples of Jesus; female as well as male apostles, and the writing out of the Feminine. This remedy may help to bring healing to schisms.

Finally there was also an entertaining reflection before the trituration began. It was noticed that before the trituration, trying to gather everyone together was difficult - everyone was off having to fix something, or do something, or had forgotten something. There was a joke about how it was like "herding cats". Everyone was off separately doing what they needed to before they were ready to come together.

Lost Generations

Given the themes of connection and separation inherent in Vesica Piscis, and that we were on stunning indigenous land in the Australian outback, it is understandable that the theme of the *Lost Generations* emerged.

Our beautiful Indigenous guide talked with us that day about some of the journey that Indigenous people have been on. Even though murder has always been illegal in Australia, a blind eye has been turned on the practice of mass poisoning of Indigenous people. In fact there was a case as recently as 1981. The land would then be taken by a white settler for grazing cattle.

We also talked about the amazing work being done by other white people to try to protect and conserve Indigenous land, the people and culture. We heard some of the beautiful examples of what Reg from Remote Education Tours, Cara and his team have been doing to help.

There are Indigenous people around the world who have separated, murdered, displaced, and the children taken, as shown in the film *Rabbit Proof Fence.*

The *Lost Generations* are, at the time of writing, yet to be a thing of the past. We see modern day human trafficking as the one of the largest illegal trades in the world. We talked quite a lot about this during this proving, along with how big corporations are part of this too and how it feels as though there is an invitation for the Divine Mother to *rise.*

We also discussed some aspects of the early sexualisation of children, and the extremes of children going to school dressed as animals, wanting trays in the toilets. We explored how this can be a move away from *knowing who we are - a separation from self,* and our true identity. One prover quoted an Ancient Greek wisdom that has been attributed to Socrates, Pythagoras and others: "Know Thyself".

My hope is that this remedy, added to the land and waters around the world, can play whatever part it can in helping reunite separated people, especially children and families, and bring healing for the lost generations.

Technology, Connection & Disconnection

During the proving, we explored the tension between modern technology (phones, internet) as a means of connection versus its role in creating disconnection or anxiety.

In this remedy is the desire to find healthier ways to connect "beyond constant digital tethering".

Bullying

Where there may be any bullying, this is a remedy that can help restore balance; there is a rebalancing of the circles, so that one is not larger than the other. There is a rebalancing of power.

There may have been an attack on the aura, this remedy can restore and heal the aura.

Shame

Brené Brown, is an academic researcher in social work, author and podcaster who has brought to our awareness what shame does in causing separation from others, and how having the courage to be vulnerable can lead to connection. Brené's 2010 TED Talk "The Power of Vulnerability" remains one of the most watched TED Talks.[37]

Shame separates us from others - from love, relationships, support, help, connection, progress.

This is a remedy for welcoming the courage to be vulnerable; to connect - to step beyond the shame that we feel and experience.

Restoration

This remedy brings restoration. This is reflected in the conversations around the wonderful work our guides are doing to restore Indigenous rights, and preserve and restore Indigenous culture.

Restoration is also present in this remedy from the reflection that this remedy was made by a Blood Wood Tree - a type of Eucalyptus that is resilient, regrows easily and sheds the resin. Blood Wood Resin is known for its glue properties - sticking things together. The tree can literally restore itself.

Grief and Loss

There is much grief and loss in the picture of this remedy, as we can imagine from the Key Themes of Separation and the Lost Generations.

As one prover said: "You are not able to have life without grief."

In the Vesica Piscis is the coming together, and so this is a remedy that calls in support through times of grief and pain so that people

37 https://www.ted.com/talks/brene_brown_the_power_of_vulnerability?utm_campaign=tedspread&utm_medium=referral&utm_source=tedcomshare

might feel less alone as they walk through it.

Homesickness

Some provers felt emotional about being far from home - especially away from their children. There was a yearning for home.

A sense of separation from home is consistent as a key note with the other themes that include separation that have been described.

Mediation

A discussion about mediation emerged - with one prover pointing out how it's remarkable to see people with "two different views, yet both working for the same thing but from different places." The prover asked the question "How do we get people to do this?".

This may be a remedy to bring people back together around a table, talking, discussing, sharing in a balanced and equal way.

Loneliness - welcomes a relationship

This is a remedy that has loneliness in its picture - the yearning for loved ones, including the yearning for a relationship if single became apparent.

This is a remedy that may help people move from feeling unattractive to connecting with their mojo. One prover talked about feeling "sexy, enticing, alluring, magnetising."

She went on to share: "Cattle station life [in Australia] means they end up wearing a lot of cattle gear. When they go into town in normal clothes it doesn't necessarily make them fanciable. In the cattle gear they can look sexy. There is a real pride in the traditional get up at rodeos, it's sexy."

One prover highlighted that "walking the path alone is a tiring process." Another felt that this is a remedy for "people who are tired of walking alone."

This may be a remedy that may help call in a significant other - the Vesica Piscis is all about moving from the one to coming together with another and forming a two!

In fact there was a lovely moment of exploring sexiness!

One prover said: "I am feeling into what it means to be sexy, enticing, alluring, magnetising. Cattle station life means that most of the time normal clothes are worn - and these clothes don't make people look particularly fanciable. However, when In the cattle gear they can look sexy. There is a real pride in the wearing of traditional gear at rodeos - and this is sexy!"

It also strikes me as significant to this key theme that the remedy was made by a Blood Wood Tree. This is a type of Eucalyptus that is resilient and can regrow easily and shed the resin. Blood Resin is good for glue properties, sticking things together.

At the time of writing, the potential for this remedy to help call in a significant other hasn't been tested, however any sharing of experiences on this would be most welcome.

Grandmothers & Amma

Several provers felt there is a grandmother energy in this remedy; the willingness of grandmothers to step forward and support the future generations. One prover connected with the protectiveness and clearing that Kali brings - the healing of the Divine Mother that comes in to clear and purify.

A beautiful conversation unfolded about Amma, who is a spiritual teacher from India who hugs thousands of people each day on the tours that she embarks upon around the world. She is said to be an *avatar.* Several of the provers had experienced *darshan* (a hug) with Amma. We reflected upon how she has built several exceptional hospitals, each has homeopathy practised within them. She donates millions to help those who experience natural disasters, war, famine. She ensures women in India are trained as plumbers so that they can build exceptional toilets for their communities, had ensured the education of millions of children, supports women to start micro-economies so that the can support themselves and their families.

Amma does more in this world to help others than any other "leader" we see, and yet many don't know about her. Her message is simple - one of love. She embodies the journey of connection - with Source, with ourselves, with our communities, with how we can serve, with love.

Staying True to Self & Sovereignty

The Vesica Piscis is made from two circles that come together equally in balance with each other. There isn't one circle that is more into the other, there is room and space for each circle to maintain it's identity, and yet each gives the same amount of themselves to create something together.

One does not subsume or consume the other.

So there is balance in the coming together, in the relationship between the circles.

We saw this reflected in the conversation that unfolded about being in relationship. As one prover said: "It's important to be true to yourself - if its not a hell yes then its a no. This is about sovereignty. It's about not trying to fit yourself into a box that does not work."

Another prover shared: "Where your aura is completely damaged, and you are trying to be your authentic self, but you are not able to express it."

Re-balancing Masculine & Feminine

There was a conversation amongst provers about how Indigenous people understand and respect gender roles. The morning of the proving, our Indigenous Guide had taken us on a beautiful walk on the land, and had told us about how there are sacred places for women where men cannot enter, and sacred places for men where women cannot enter.

Our Guide taught us about how Indigenous Australians understand that the mother teaches the child. Everyone has their place. The child is raised in the early years by the mother and the feminine line. We were shown a beautiful birthing cave, however only women are allowed to enter. Men do not cross a line to enter it, they are respectful.

As one prover said: "The indigenous people worldwide - when the white man conquered the lands, with their own rules, and with being heavily male dominated, in cultures where females and males had their own rules, this changed. There was a shift in the role of the female and that division has filtered down to the Indigenous people. The females had their [important] roles, and this changed when the white men came, women then took more of a back seat."

There was a reflection of how similar this is in some other cultures; a respecting of natural lore.

There was also an exploration of the masculine / feminine and how it is represented in the Christian church, and how there were both female and male Apostles; which is completely aligned with what is conventionally understood about the Essences; the tribe that Jesus was both into. One prover stated that: "The Christian church does not have the feminine mystical. This remedy has that."

Success, harmony & balance

In the same way that there is an invitation to return to a re-balancing of the masculine and feminine, and that there is equal space and room for both, this is a remedy that invites the same in terms of what success looks like.

Capitalist models place money and numbers at the centre of life - and success is measured by having the highest numbers. This however as we discussed often comes at a price; compromised quality, the inability to drop as deeply into something and a often a lack of consideration for whether this is in balance with nature.

I was reminded of a teaching by Francesca Mason Boring, a remarkable teacher who I was blessed to be taught by when studying to become a Family Constellations Facilitator. Francesca has Indigenous American ancestry. She described how Indigenous cultures place meaning and connection at the centre of life. Keeping a connection to higher wisdom and knowledge ensures there is always a balance with nature in life. The Western world places materialism at the centre of life, and this creates distortion and a lack of balance.

There was a conversation around what balance looks like - ensuring that there is room for everyone, in balance and harmony. As Gandhi said: "There is enough for everyone's need not everyone's greed."

A further conversation centred around corporations creating products with "manufacturing obsolescence" - particularly where this is planned by companies in order that people keep buying from them. One prover said: "I amazingly have a boiler in my home that is 45 years old, working perfectly well. It is almost completely mechanical, and so there aren't electrical parts that could cause it to stop working. Plumbers love coming to service it because they say it's so rare to get to see one!".

Other conversations around corporate greed centred around the poisoning of water supplies by companies, for example as depicted in the movies *Erin Brokovich* and *Dark Waters.*

The Vesica Piscis recognises the true definitions of success, and this remedy restores balance to how we relate to what success truly is, a realigning with there being enough for everyone.

There is also a reminder in this remedy of how success has come to meant in Western ideology living in your home, separate to parents, and it used to be a sign of financial success. Current economic structures mean that increasing numbers of younger people are remaining living at home with their parents for longer, as younger generations cannot afford to buy their own homes. This used to be a source of shame, but this is changing.

As one prover said: "Covid made it easier. So many lost their jobs, income and livelihoods then, and there was only compassion showed to those that had a change in their income. We all lost a layer of shame in talking about having or not having money - it was an unintended consequence of Covid. Also, children are now having to live with their parents for longer, going back to tribal living structures. We are returning to or staying with our village."

Simplicity

This remedy returns us to a state of remembering what truly matters and feels aligned; there is a gratitude for the simple things in life.

As one prover shared: "This remedy helps us to return to what helps us feel connected - to our families, friendships, to nature, life, each other."

Clarity

This is a remedy that - when puzzled and confused - it will bring clarity in a gentle way. As one prover shared: "masterting the mundane, master what steps need to be taken one by one, and the bigger picture will fall into place."

Where we feel separated from our next steps, solutions, our ability to find a way forward and make decisions, this is a remedy that can help us to connect with them once more.

Time

It allows time to stretch back and forth in plenty of time, just really subtle and trust the process.

There is a recognition of "Divine Timing" in this remedy; how everything happens in its own (right) time, and cannot be forced. One prover said "we can try a few different ways to make something work once the grain of sand starts that allows things to follow but you cannot force that. It takes time. Like an hourglass."

There is also an invitation in this remedy to connect with timelessness; the experience that children have when they play, when they lose all sense of time. This is a remedy that returns a balance of time, and being able to be present and aligned with it.

The Vesica Piscis is not the same as the infinity symbol, and yet they are not entirely unlike each other. In the infinity symbol, there is a constant flow and movement, with the Vescia Piscis there is a birthing or emerging of something new from the bringing together of different aspects through time and space.

Post Natal Depression, Mother & Child Bonding, Issues affecting women & parents

When we look at the Vesica Piscis, we also see the vulva represented. The coming together of two separate aspects through which a third can be birthed.

This is a remedy that can really support women through some of the challenges that women can face.

Post-natal depression can, according to some research, be caused by the sudden drop in progesterone following birth. Other risk factors include separation from people or land of origin, having been bereaved of one or both parents, being unsupported, being in an unloving relationship. HPA (hypothalamus-pituitary-adrenal) axis dysregulation can also be a risk factor - which can have been caused by traumatic life events.[38] All of these factors can contribute

38Yim IS, Tanner Stapleton LR, Guardino CM, Hahn-Holbrook J, Dunkel Schetter C. Biological and psychosocial predictors of postpartum depression: systematic review

to difficulties in mother and baby bonding - which is another expression of separation; how can a mother who isn't held herself then hold the life that come through her? How can a mother who is unsupported then support the life that has come through her?

Other situations affecting women where this remedy may help is:

- Hormonal imbalances (separation from a balance of what gives us power as women)
- Birth trauma
- Miscarriages
- Endometriosis
- Fibroids
- All issues to do with the womb
- Women facing a hysterectomy (separation from the main organ that defines us as women)
- Mother-child bonding difficulties (separation from each other)
- Parents experiencing parental alienation or separation from their child
- Empty nest syndrome

Vision

When we look at the Vesica Piscis, we can see the eye. The eye brings together all the information it can gather, and from all the information gathered, a decision is made about next steps; the expression (or birthing) of a new step.

There is an aspect of the Vesica Piscis that includes and involves the bringing together the different aspects of a vision so that it can be materialised or manifested into form.

---

and call for integration. Annu Rev Clin Psychol. 2015;11:99-137. doi: 10.1146/annurev-clinpsy-101414-020426. PMID: 25822344; PMCID: PMC5659274

Mental & Emotional Symptoms

Feeling lonely
Feeling tired of walking alone
Resilience and endurance
Deep grief and division; grief is unavoidable
Grief better consolation
Empty nest syndrome
Mother-child bonding difficulties
Imbalance of masculine / feminine
Children who do not get through life without grief
Feeling panicky
Claustrophobia
Overwhelming fear
Dependence on technology creating anxiety and disconnection
Emotional cords cutting
Bullying
Trying to be authentic but unable to express self
Separation and division causing shame and distancing from family & loved ones
Feeling overwhelmed and tired of walking alone
Loneliness but being okay with it
Busy mind
Difficulties being able to relax
Shame around cultural boundaries and fitting in
Shame
Resilience and endurance
Mastering the mundane
Trusting the process
Corporate exploitation
Anxiety around modern identity and confusion
Unsure how to take the next step
Lack of support
Expressing desires
Balance of material and spiritual

Lack of sovereignty
Confusion

Physical Particular Symptoms

Head

Throbbing on one side of head (either side)

Eyes

Eye injury
Visual impairment
Difficulties seeing
One eye larger than the other
One pupil larger than the other

Ears

No direct mention of ear symptoms; mention of trouble hearing and taking energy

Throat

Needing to express desires

Lungs & Breathing

Difficulties with inspiration
Constricted breathing

Heart

Pericardium damage

Digestion

SIBO
Candida

Bladder

Water imbalances
Oedema

Female Reproductive

Hormonal imbalances
Birth trauma
Miscarriages
Endometriosis
Fibroids
Womb lining
Uterine problems
Birth - cervix not opening

Physical General Symptoms

Sleep

Feeling sleepy
Overactive mind preventing sleep

Dreams

Dreams of young children

Food & Drink

Eating too much processed foods

Energy Levels

Fatigue
Doing bare minimum needed to complete tasks
Tired of walking alone

Clinical

All issues relating to female reproduction
Any situation where there is an imbalance between paired organs; where one of a paired organ is working better/worse than the other
Candida
SiBO

Spiritual

Connection with Egypt, pyramid
Isis
Spiritual healing remedies; subtlety and purity in remedy making
Connection with Gaia and need for reconnecting to Earth
Schism in Christianity and loss of feminine mystical energy
Indigenous worldwide history of female/male roles and their shift
Returning to tribal living structures; governed by soul and natural lore
Calling in mother energy, Divine Mother, Grandmothers, and feminine healing
Amma
Spiritual service
Remedy to bring relationships and partnership
Psychic cords and spiritual connection beyond physical technology

Feeling of being "home" wherever one goes; connection to land and family
Healing trauma through plant and natural energies
Divine timing and trusting process
Energy of magnetic forces and coming together
The seed resembling a brain, aligning hemispheres
Awareness of integrity over social media or superficial measures
Healing of the Divine Mother birthing the fire of the feminine
"Be the change you want to see" - Gandhi

Remedy Affinities

Aluminium
Ambra grisea
Anacardium
Aurum metallicum
Aurum muriaticum
Bay Leaf
Chesnut white
Dodona
Carcinosin
Goldfish
Lac Caninum
Lac Humanum
Lycopodium
Nux vomica
Oxytocin
Petrified Sequoia
Phosphoricum acidum
Platina
Staphysagria
Tarentula
Thuja
Thymus gland
Viscum album

The Seed of Life

14 August 2025
Lilla
Watarrka Land
Northern Territory
Australia

This trituration took place on 14 August 2025, at Lilla, a stunning indigenous outstation in Wattarka National Park in Central Australia. The remedy was made two days following the Venus-Jupiter conjunction that had peaked on 12 August. Venus, the planet of love, beauty, and harmony, joined Jupiter, the planet of expansion, abundance, and wisdom bringing an energy of love, abundance, and optimism.

7 provers were involved with this trituration, all 7 were women. This was triturated using the intuitive trituration method to a 13c.

The Seed of Life

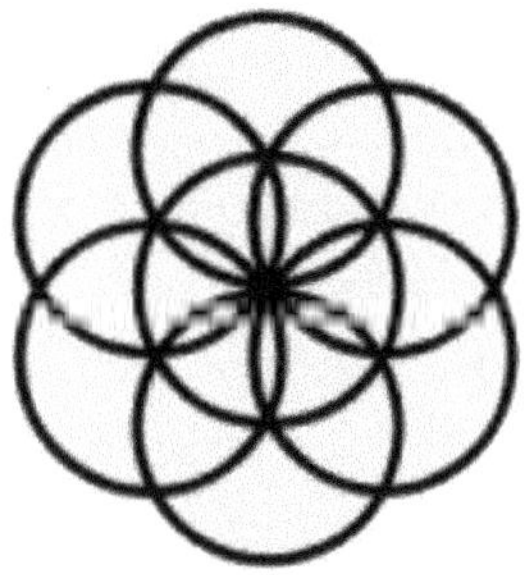

The Seed of Life consists of 7 circles that overlap & represents the 7 days of creation. It is the seed of the Flower of Life. The Seed of Life connects with how life starts from a seed, and then blossoms and grows – just like the universe has done. It also corresponds to exactly how a 3 day old embryo looks - the point at which it becomes a multicellular organism.)

Each of the 7 circles overlaps with and shares it's centre with others, and so is also considered to reflect how all things are interconnected.

Seed of Life Homeopathic Remedy™

Key Themes

Growth, Fertility & Renewal
Potential & Possibility
Communication, Connection & Care for Others
Stem Cells
Manifestation / Materialisation
Vibrancy & Regeneration
Children
Transformation & Change
Beauty and Self-worth
Cycles of Life & Initiations
Time

Growth, Fertility & Renewal

Seeds grow in darkness, just like babies in the womb. The Seed of Life returns us to that void space where there is so much potential for growth and expansion. As one prover said;

"There is a theme of darkness - the light form is created, the seed. What is planted underneath needs too be hidden and stay away from the middle earth, in order to keep it sacred and keep the life form growing. It brings with it anticipation and excitement and also this knowing that you are not able to stay in that place, knowing that change needs to happen and with that transformation."

Potential & Possibility

The Seed of Life connects us with potential and possibility. There is within this a choice. As one prover said: "This remedy is like entering a museum where you can experience all the stages of evolution, as you go back through time. You might see a tree and then you go back to the root. This is about going back to the root, back to the potential from which it is possible to go that way or this way but there is choice in this remedy." As another prover said "Alternating realities, what if I had chosen the other route, what would have transpired?"

There was another interesting connection with potential; in how there is the potential to connect with every other part of the body through the feet, as seen in reflexology maps of the feet. Fractals of connection.

Potential was also explored in relation to meeting individual needs. "There are different methods of parenting, diets, nothing is relevant, it should be a personalised approach. Trends are common, but in the context of supplements, sometimes they can be dangerous [if not what a person actually needs]".

Communication, Connection & Care for Others

The experience of potential extends into the potential with other people. One prover described the remedy as having a "potential for dialogue, different concepts, this space where you are able to have conversations, real collaboration and elaboration, non-attachment and meeting in the middle ground."

True potential takes in all possibilities. As another prover shared: "Communication is about listening to what is said and what is not said."

There was a considerable amount of caring between members of the group. Different members reached out to help, support or care for others. The care was given easily, and from a place of balance; it felt natural and easy to give. One prover for example was finding it difficult to get comfortable, and so another member started to massage her back. Another shared a drink. Yet another wanted to place her feet in water, so another prover arranged this.

Stem Cells

It was found that this remedy "works at a cellular level.". This is a remedy that connects us with stem cells; cells that have the potential to differentiate into different tissues, organs and structures of the body.

This potential is so beautifully described by Dr Bruce Lipton, a cell biologist and researcher at Stanford University who conducted very interesting research on stem cells.

He took cloned stem cells and placed them in 3 different Petri dishes, each containing a slightly different culture medium.

The cells were genetically identical - yet in one dish, the cells became muscle. In another, they became bone. In the third they became fat cells.

The only difference for the cells was the environment that they found themselves in. Dr Lipton equates this to what is circulating in the blood - that the blood is like the culture medium in the Petri dish.

What is the blood being flooded with? Neurotransmitters and hormones that are secreted in response to how we think and feel.

Dr Lipton says: "In my lectures, I simply give this story:

If you are sitting there with your eyes closed and you open your eyes and see someone you love, your mind holds a picture of love. A picture of love in the mind is translated by the brain into very specific chemistry. In a state of love, the brain releases dopamine for pleasure into the blood. The brain releases oxytocin into the blood, which is a chemical that helps us bind to the source of love that we are experiencing. The experience of love also releases another chemical into the growth medium—into the blood—called vasopressin. It helps us become more attractive so that our partner sticks with us even more. Another very important factor released by our brain while perceiving love is growth hormone—which, by its name does exactly what it says: It influences our growth. That result is that the chemistry of the body's natural culture medium—blood—is adjusted by the perception of the mind.

The perception of love introduces such elements as dopamine, oxytocin, vasopressin, and growth hormone, all of which are chemicals that enhance the vitality and health of the 50 trillion cells in our skin-covered culture dish. In a state of love, the chemicals released in love result in health and harmony and a glowing body. People say, "Oh, look, you can see how in love they are. See how they glow." That is a chemical expression of the culture medium, affecting the vitality of the cells.

Then I say, "Wait. The same person could open their eyes and instead of seeing love, see something that scares them." In a state of fear, the brain does not release the chemicals associated with love. It releases chemicals associated with fear, which are stress hormones and inflammatory agents, changing the chemistry of the culture medium. Then, go back and recognise that the fate of the cell is directly dependent on the chemistry of the culture medium.

Now with stress hormones and inflammatory agents released in the blood, I change the genetics and behaviour of the cells and start to express a protection posture, which is antagonistic to growth. In fact, it actually cancels growth. The protection chemicals in the blood allocate energy for fight or flight, getting ready to run from a perceived fear."[39]

Our emotions and beliefs contribute to the expression of our cells and how they develop. This is a remedy that connects us with that potential.

Manifestation / Materialisation

During the proving, we connected with the Ascended Master Melchizedek, who represents manifestation. Manifestation is considered in some schools of thinking to be the masculine form of the word (hence "man" as the root of the word), whereas materialisation is the feminine form of the word - the root of this word is mater (Latin for "mother"). It is the mother that can literally bring into material form a child that she dreamed of.

This is a remedy that helps with both.

Vibrancy & Regeneration

Any seed contains potential - and when this is realised, it has an energy of vibrancy. One prover described the remedy as having a "warmth - warming things up, bringing things back to life - vibrancy. Another prover stated that the remedy is connected to: "start of life stuff but this remedy is also for the elderly to bring vibrancy, brings back vibrancy." Another prover described a "reset, restart, rejuvenation". Yet another described how every day she says to herself: "I am totally regenerating myself."

This is a remedy that brings regeneration.

---

39 Gustafson C. Bruce Lipton, PhD: The Jump From Cell Culture to Consciousness. Integr Med (Encinitas). 2017 Dec;16(6):44-50. PMID: 30936816; PMCID: PMC6438088

Children

This is a remedy for children. One of the provers was 36 weeks pregnant at the time of the proving, and felt her baby moving around much more than usual.

The remedy's ability to connect us with potential is also another way in which this remedy can be good for children.

Transformation & Change

We have already touched upon the theme of the seed growing in the darkness, unseen, and so we see transformation and change - this is what the potential in this remedy enables; new possibilities unfolding.

Beauty and Self-Worth

This remedy connects us with the beauty in everything, from beauty at a "skin-deep" level, through all the layers of a person's being.

We were reminded of a story that one of the provers had heard of how confused the people in an African tribe had been at being invited to consider whether they thought themselves to be beautiful. They didn't understand the context, so the visitors explained that many people, especially women, in Western cultures could not perceive their own beauty. The African tribespeople were shocked by this, for they have an innate understanding that each person is beautiful, and they never question this within themselves.

This is a remedy that connects us with the perfection and beauty within us and in all of life. In this way, it has an affinity with Thuja.

One prover had, in fact, had a dream just before about a child with a Thuja tree. "I had a dream where a 4-5 year old said he has a Thuja tree and loves it and that night I saw a human version of the remedy in the dream."

Cycles of Life & Initiations

The cycles of life, birth, fertility, and death were explored during the proving. Ovulation cycles were also reflected upon; it feels again as though this is a connection to potential.

This may be a remedy to use alongside others during detoxification of synthetic hormones, as it connects us with natural cycles of life.

Discussions around initiations, and how we know that we moving from one time in our lives to another. One prover shared an initiation practice used by one of the Indigenous peoples of Anangu. To be able to move from one time period, or state, into another is to move into new possibilities and express an unfolding potential.

We discussed how an understanding and appreciation of this has been lost in Western cultures. This is a remedy that helps us to connect with those necessary cycles, initiations and transitions.

Time

All of the sacred geometry remedies have a same common theme with that of time. With the Seed of Life, it was found in body rhythms, pregnancy, and the unfolding time needed for natural processes to take place.

Mental & Emotional Symptoms

Feeling self-contained
Feeling very tired, exhausted
Communication: listening, dialogue, non-attachment, meeting in the middle ground
For where there is a lack of appreciation of one's own beauty, or beauty in the surroundings - this remedy welcomes that appreciation of beauty
Difficulties expressing emotion - welcomes the beauty in being free with emotion
Feel shut down
Bullying
Phobias, fears
Parents unsure about how to approach parenting their child - helps parents find a personalised approach to raising their child
Serenity in this remedy - welcomes a feeling that it is okay just to be
Cannot see any way out - opens to new potentials and possibilities
Lack of self-care - welcomes an understanding of own needs

Physical Particulars

Head

Headache on left side coming down towards neck, sharp pain
Headache on left side and shoulder slightly
Headache has gone

Ears

Hearing not the best at the moment, helps with hearing

Nose

Sniffly and depleted, viral infection-like symptoms
Congestion

Lungs & Breathing

Sudden congestion in lungs

Digestion

Constipation, clears bowels

Female Reproduction

Clearing synthetic hormones
Fertility
Ovulation
Irregular menses

Male Reproduction

Erectile dysfunction
Problems with testicles
Increasing sperm vitality and motility
Testosterone imbalance

Back & Limbs

Fungal toe nails
Restless legs
Weak bones

Skin

Warts
Insect bites and stings
Mosquito bites
Fungal toe nails
Ringworm

Physical Generals

Sleep

Sleep talking

Dreams

Of trees and nature

Body Temperature

A good fever remedy
Sensitive to cold and chilly winds
Brings warmth

Food & Drink

Craving for chocolate

Energy Levels

Feeling tired, depleted, exhausted
Vibrancy returning, brings back life
Brings a reset, restart, rejuvenation

Clinical

Viral infections
This remedy works at a cellular level
Chicken pox
Cold, flu symptoms
Remedy for metabolic disorders
Osteoporosis (in combination with other remedies eg symphytum)

Spiritual

Fire symbolism: transformation, sacredness, ceremonies
Connection with Melchizedek - Ascended master - and manifestation / materialisation / spiritual connection
Wishes and beauty
Symbolism of the Divine Feminine
Indigenous initiation rituals

Remedy Affinities

Ash
Aurum
Butterfly
Calc phos
Carbo veg
Carcinosin
Golden Spiral
Phosphorus
Platina
Silver birch
Symphytum
Thuja

Egg of Life

11 August 2025
Alice Springs
Northern Territory
Australia

This trituration took place on 11 August 2025 in the lead up to a Venus-Jupiter conjunction that peaked on 12 August. Venus, the planet of love, beauty, and harmony, joined Jupiter, the planet of expansion, abundance, and wisdom bringing an energy of love, abundance, and optimism.

7 provers were involved with this trituration, all 7 were women. This was triturated using the intuitive trituration method to a 13c.

The Egg of Life

The Egg of Life represents the stage of growth of the embryo when it has divided into 4 and then into 8 cells; these 8 spheres make up the sacred geometry of the Egg of Life. The Seed of Life represents pure potential, whereas with the Egg of Life we have crossed into the actual realisation of that potential in physical form.

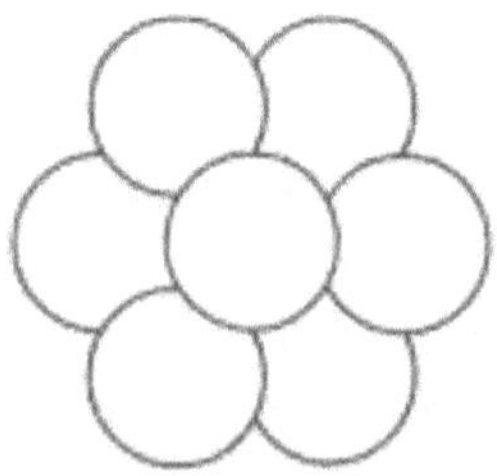

The Egg of Life represents fertility, and also cell division.

We see the number 8 here: this is the number of the octave, which connects us with *Harmonia,* as Pythagoras taught us. It is also a number of power and transformation, which is relevant to the cells being able to transform from this state into what is needed.

Egg of Life Homeopathic Remedy™

Key Themes

Feminine Power
Fertility
Reverence for the Mother
Visibility
Creation
Ancestral Healing
Cosmic Origins
Grief
Regret
Divine Timing
Time

Feminine Power

The Egg of Life supports the reclamation of feminine wisdom and power. This includes all that is held within the womb, as well as supporting fertility, pregnancy, menstruation, and birth in sacred and powerful ways.

One prover became excited describing the recent scientific discoveries that the human egg chooses the sperm that fertilises her - which has been a significant reversal of conventional narratives, and has reminded us of the power of feminine autonomy.

This is a remedy to also consider for the suppression of feminine power. During the proving we discussed how the power of the feminine is suppressed through the use of birth control and patriarchal systems that have literally written women out of being seen as important as men.

Our hormones are messengers within the body, communicating what needs to happen in order for us to stay healthy and well. Every part of our physical body has an energetic or quantum aspect to it - and so our hormones are not only messengers within the body, but without too, they also connect with and communicate with the cosmos. We see this in how women's hormones are influenced by the phases of the moon. These phases move through cycles that enhance our intuition, guide us to take action and invite us to rest at different times.

Synthetic contraceptive hormones take over control of and literally flatline the natural ebb and flow of our hormonal cycles - what we need in order to have a truly enhanced intuition. It is our intuition that makes us powerful as women. And so synthetic hormones suppress feminine power.

Another prover described the power that we have as women to choose whether we fall pregnant at all. She recalled: "I fell pregnant at a time when it wasn't alright for me to have a child. I was in the very early stages, but already my body had begun to change. So I sat down one evening, and spoke to the soul. I thanked it for coming to me. I explained that I was full of love and gratitude, but that now wasn't the right time for me to be able to provide the little one with all it needed for a wonderful life, which is what it deserved. So I thanked it and asked it to leave my body. The next morning I bled through."

Women were said once upon a time to have the power to choose consciously when they fell pregnant and with whom, but that this power has been forgotten.

Another prover said: "It connects us with choice, trusting in the bigger picture, for when we cannot see in the moment that our power is within us, it is not external. It connects us with Divine timing. There is this other sense of when you materialise a miracle in your life - we've all experienced miracles in some way shape or form.....you can't put into words the feelings. It's elation, more than joy, more than happiness, it's up there. This is a bridge remedy, it connects us - physically, but in a very present way - like thymus gland, it is at the beginning but it carries forward, moving quickly."

The themes in this remedy were very much a reconnection with the innate power of the feminine, with the sacredness of the feminine, and a moving beyond how the feminine has been controlled.

We were reminded of the power of the egg choosing the sperm, a fact that has only relatively recently come to light. Research published by Fitzpatrick et al in the Journal of the Proceedings of the Royal Society in 2020 demonstrated this. The researchers think that the egg sends out chemical signals that have been named chemoattractants to attract the sperm she likes and slows down the rest. Specific sperm are thought by this research to be chosen based on genetic compatibility. Furthermore, eggs can influence the sperm that reach them, even if the sperm don't belong to the woman's partner.[40]

This is another example of the connection with feminine power.

It is a wonderful remedy to give alongside synthetic hormone detoxes (please also see prescribing notes).

Fertility

It addresses physical, emotional, and energetic blocks in relation to fertility, including blocked fallopian tubes, fibroids, cysts, hormonal

40 John L. Fitzpatrick, Charlotte Willis, Alessandro Devigili, Amy Young, Michael Carroll, Helen R. Hunter, Daniel R. Brison; Chemical signals from eggs facilitate cryptic female choice in humans. Proc Biol Sci 1 June 2020; 287 (1928): 20200805

imbalances, the influence of birth control pills and trauma.

There is a call to birthing new possibilities with this remedy,

Reverence for the Mother

This remedy brings deep reverence for **the mother**, both archetypal and physical.

Visibility

Some provers felt a connection with presence and visibility with this remedy.

Creation

As well as a reconnection to the power of the feminine, this is a remedy that supports creative processes, and the sacredness and seriousness of creation.

As we have already seen, this is a remedy that connects us with the deep intuitive knowing of what and when to create in relation to fertility.

The stories of creation also emerged during the proving. As one prover said:

"The Indigenous people of these lands [Australia where the remedy was triturated] get the stars, the importance of the stars, how everything is aligned with the stars, how every dream, every intention cannot be if not aligned with the stars. We have forgotten our roots, where we came from. We came from the heavens - not via genesis [Adam and Eve] or having evolved from monkeys. The true creation story is from the stars, without them we are nothing, they write and weave the stories of our creation, the very fabric of who we are".

In order for creation to be possible, coherence is necessary. As one prover described it, "synchronised across different realms, this remedy brings it all into sync; coherence."

Ancestral Healing

Our cells carry the memories, experiences and of course miasmatic influences of our ancestors. This was felt very much with this remedy.

Here we have a connection with fossil remedies - people needing fossil remedies may carry a sense of the ancestral or karmic past; problems that feel like they span generations or even lifetimes.

Cosmic Origins

There was a recognition and celebration of how indigenous peoples understand the importance of the stars, how everything is aligned with the stars, and how every dream and intention cannot be if not aligned with the stars.

As one prover said "remembering this is necessary and needed for health on our planet. We have forgotten our roots and where we came from. We came from the heavens. We have been conventionally taught only two origin stories; that there was either Genesis, and that we came from Adam and Eve..... or that we evolved from primates according to Charles Darwin's Theory of Evolution. The true origin story is that we came from the stars, but this was written out. The stars write and weave the stories of our creation, the very fabric of who we are."

Grief

Deep grief is one of the key themes of this remedy - especially grief that is connected to the feminine, or grief for not having been able to create a wish or a desire. One prover said:

"I am feeling a grief, deep, old grief that I didn't still know was in my body, mind and soul. Deep grief of the heart, regret. I have been remembering painful times from when I was a teenager, and home wasn't a safe space for me.....I have been crying remembering those times, and feeling sorrow about how I wasn't able to create the life of my dreams a young child. I was bereft. I wasn't safe. I couldn't create the life of my dreams. I was surrounded by wealthy, rich pupils and their families, and their nice houses and normal family lives, with a Mum and a Dad, and it felt like another world away from my own life. I couldn't connect to it, it wasn't my life."

Another prover said:

"I am reminded of my dear friend. She is DESPERATE for another child. She is pining for the other child she wished she could have had. Part of it is because she looks back and sees the mother that she was for her first child as one that wasn't really there all the time for her child, she was a young mother, and not ready for it, not always as patient as she wishes she could have been. She would love to have the experience of having another child now - with all of the lessons, the calm, the peacefulness, presence, patience that she is able to give a child. She is full of regret, and sorrow. She is desperate to create the life she wished she could have had."

Regret

In this remedy is regret as well as grief; regret for how their life has not worked out the way they had wanted it to, regretting not being able to create the life they would have wished to be able to do.

One prover was remembering a time from a childhood. She said: "I have been remembering the challenges during my teenage years, even though it was decades ago. I have been crying remembering those times, and feeling sorrow about how I wasn't able to create the life of my dreams as a young child. I was bereft. I wasn't safe. I was surrounded by wealthy, rich girls and their families, and their nice houses and normal family lives, with a Mum and a Dad, and it felt like another world away from my own life. I couldn't connect to it, it wasn't my life."

Another said "I am reminded of a friend who is desperate for another child. She is pining for the other child she wished she could have had. Part of it is because she looks back and sees the mother that she was as one that wasn't ready for it, not always as patient as she wishes she could have been. She would love another child to have the experience of having one now - with all of the lessons, the calm, the peacefulness, presence, patience that she is able to give a child. She is full of regret, and sorrow. She is desperate to create the life she wished she could have had."

Divine Timing

This remedy welcomes a connection with, and remembrance of Diving Timing. There is an invitation to trust in the bigger picture of life.

Time

This is a remedy that connects us with time. There is a timeless quality to it.

It also welcomes a slowing down. As one prover experienced: "There is no time to waste, we've got to keep moving forward. Hurried lives, where we do not know how to slow down. This brings balance to the forces of time moving in all directions and brings us closer to that still point in the centre of the yin yang."

As we have seen, the Egg of Life has some alignment with fossil themes, including supporting those who feel "frozen in time" emotionally or psychologically. This, of course, can also have an impact on flow, and fertility and creation.

Mental / Emotional Symptoms

Regret for not creating the life one dreamed of
Deep grief
Sorrow from feeling unsafe in childhood
Desperation for a child
Desire for redemption as a mother
Regret as a mother
Grief about missed motherhood opportunities
Feeling unlovable, unwanted
Feeling invisible
Personal fakery, not authentic
Despair and suppression
Control issues, patriarchy
Forgetfulness, struggle with learning
Mocking energy; having been bullied

Women dismissed or not listened to
Fear of revealing incapacity
Desperation to create meaning
Innocence and need to be held
Not seeing in the moment
Seeing people's defects; judgement
Grief stored in the lungs
Desire to express innate power
Emotional recall of teenage trauma
Deep grief of the heart
Song: "Sweet Disposition"
Sovereignty & individuation

Physical Particular Symptoms

Ears

Sound of bells ringing

Nose

Hyper-acute sense of smell
Smell of sugar

Throat

Suppression of voice / not being heard

Lungs & Breathing

Grief is often stored in lungs

Digestion

Constipation
Nausea
Stomach

Physical gut-level grief or shock

Liver

Excess oestrogen from environment
Hormonal imbalance, possible liver load

Female Reproductive

Fibroids
Cysts
Spot on left cheek – hormonal/oestrogen
Oestrogen excess
Prolapsed cervix
Poor quality eggs
Bleeding out
Unwanted pregnancy - helps align with choices and next steps
On the pill – suppression
Suppression of fertility by chemical/human/emotional barrier
Feminine energy, emits power
Women not in control; patriarchy illusion
Excess oestrogen from environment
Hormonal imbalance

Male Reproduction

Supports egg choosing sperm

Back & Limbs

Dyspraxia
Awkwardness
Clumsiness
Poor co-ordination

Physical General Symptoms

Sleep

Difficulty sleeping fully through the night

Dreams

Caring for a child
Caring for a disabled child
Unconditional love
Remembering forgotten origins, dreams of alignment with the stars

Food & Drink

Smell of sugar; agg.

Energy Levels

Hurried, fast-paced energy
Need to keep moving forward
Speedy

Clinical

Infertility (male and female)
Hormone imbalances

Spiritual

Ancestors coming through
Offering to humanity
Reverence and sacredness of pregnancy
Conscious creation
Power of remembering
Feminine creation energy suppressed
Importance of stars, alignment, origins
Star beings
Synchronisation across realms
Sitting in a circle in another realm
Flower of Life, Neolithic goddess traditions

Remedy Affinities

All Matridonal & Lac Remedies
Ayahuasca
Chalice Well Water
Chestnut red
Fruit of Life
Folliculinum
Lac Maternum
Metatron's Cube
Milky Way
Moonstone
Nat mur
Olive
Petrified Sequoia
Phosphorus
Pituitary Gland
Pleiades
Red
Sandalwood
Sea salt

Silver birch
Thuja
Vesica Piscis

Prescribing Notes

1. This remedy can be given alongside hormone detoxes, particularly where there are plans to try to conceive.

Fruit of Life

12 August 2025
Palm Valley
Cycad Gorge
Northern Territory
Australia

This trituration took place on 12 August 2025 during the peak of the Venus-Jupiter conjunction. Venus, the planet of love, beauty, and harmony, joined Jupiter, the planet of expansion, abundance, and wisdom bringing an energy of love, abundance, and optimism.

7 provers were involved with this trituration, all 7 were women. This was triturated using the intuitive trituration method to a 13c.

The Fruit of Life

The Fruit of Life is composed of 13 spheres. 13 represents unity & connection through dimensions & worlds. In a chromatic scale of 12 notes, there is a 13 - it's the same note as the first, but another octave higher, representing moving into a higher dimension.

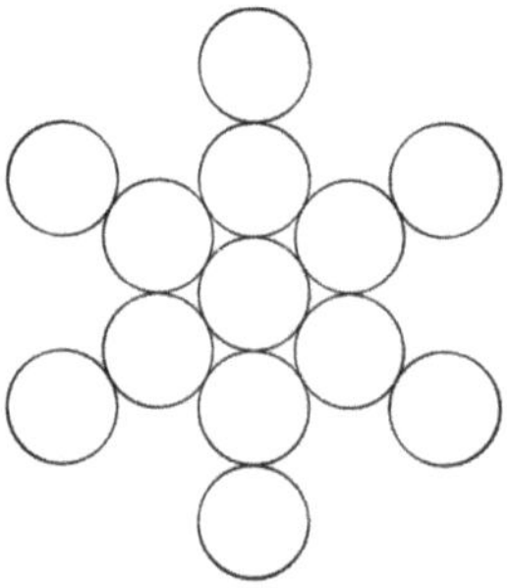

13 is also the number of the Divine Feminine; there are 13 moons in a calendar year, and so 13 menstrual (lunar) cycles for women whose cycles are 28 days long.. In Ancient Egypt, 13 represented the joyous afterlife.

The Fruit of Life encourages us to move towards our desires & goals; turning our aspirations into a reality, just like the Divine Feminine materialises what is a desire into physical material form in order to become mothers.

Fruit of Life Homeopathic Remedy™

Key Themes

Death (as transformation)
New beginnings
Stillness
Reproduction
Sacred Masculine & Sacred Feminine
Body acceptance
Connection with Nature - especially Bees
Vision
Cosmic & Body Cycles

Death (as transformation)

We were told a very powerful story by our guide about meeting Death. In the telling of the story was a great respect for Death, and also, for the experience of recognising when it is and isn't time for passing.

The Fruit of Life, as we have already written connects us with the number 13 and how, In a chromatic scale of 12 notes, there is a 13 - it's the same note as the first, but another octave higher, representing moving into a higher dimension.

In order to move into the next octave, there is a leaving behind of the previous octave; a moving into a higher dimension. This is a death to the old, and a birth to the new.

A mother when she is birthing her first child is also experiencing a death; a death to the time of being a maiden. The baby, being birthed into a new life, is leaving behind the time of being in spirit, and then being in the womb, to emerge into a new life; a new world.

During the proving, we could hear ravens and crows. Both of these birds symbolise death and transformation as well as messages from spirit.

A miscarriage that a prover had experienced kept coming up, there were recollections of partners, pets and loved ones that had died.

This remedy can bring an understanding of and acceptance of and respect for the purpose of death. It is not so much a grief remedy per se, as it is an invitation to understand and come to acceptance around death.

New beginnings

13 is the same note as the first in a chromatic scale of 12 notes, but another octave higher, representing moving into a higher dimension. Or a birth into new beginnings!

The new beginnings are not just in relation to physical birth, and the emergence into the world; but also with conception itself. Several provers discussed experiencing a connection with conception.

One prover said: "There is a rebirth, shedding, stillness, letting go. Whatever is holding us back, we are letting that go, and moving into new spaces."

Stillness

At birth and at death, there is a deep experience of stillness; as if all time has converged into this single moment - or as if there is a stillness as the portals between worlds open as souls arrive or depart.

There was a deep and profound stillness during this proving; a deep calm and peace settled on the whole group that mirrored that point of transformation.

The stillness brought with it a deep grounding - and a connection with what is true; something that becomes very clear at times of transition.

Where there is too much life stress, it was found that this remedy brings us back to stillness, and to nature.

Reproduction

All aspects of female reproduction are supported by the Fruit of Life; healthy menstruation, conception, pregnancy, menopause. All imbalance in the cycles and physiology of women were discussed in relation to this remedy.

This is also a remedy to help improve men's sperm.

Blood

Menstruation, menopause, first bleeds and blood rituals were all discussed. One peri-menopausal prover had begun her first bleed in nine months. Clots were also discussed, as well as a lack of blood flow.

The importance of iron was also discussed - how iron is needed both to birth a baby and for healthy blood.

Sacred Masculine & Sacred Feminine

In order for the sacred feminine to flow, to create, to allow life to move through her, the sacred masculine needs to hold space for this to happen.

This is a remedy for both the masculine and feminine; it helps to invite a space holding that the masculine can do in order that the feminine can flow and create.

Dr Zach Bush teaches that "the role of the masculine is to see the beauty in the feminine", and this is very relevant to the relationship between the sacred masculine and sacred feminine, along with another key theme of this remedy; body acceptance.

There was a very beautiful moment when three of the women provers decided to swim naked in a pool in the stunning gorge before the trituration. The one man present respectfully took himself away, as though he were beautifully holding space for us to do so.

One prover found herself needing to move, and experienced this as an expanding; a move into the space as a woman, where she was allowed to occupy and take ownership of the space.

This remedy connects with Goddess energy, especially Isis. It is a remedy that is closely linked to the remedy Dodona.

There was also a deeply profound moment in the day when the one man who was with us shared some of his own experiences and inner self. During the trituration, we reflected on this, and our deep respect for him. It felt like a deeply healing connection, and that he was holding our circle so beautifully, and with great tenderness.

We reflected on intimacy. This is a remedy that can connect us with

intimacy once more.
The song "Sweet Disposition" by The Temper Trap was a theme that day for two of the provers, having heard it played in a shop en route to the gorge. The song is about the exhilarating, innocent, and often fleeting feeling of young love, youthful freedom, and embracing a moment of pure connection, which felt very relevant to the themes of this proving.

Body acceptance

Body acceptance is a key theme in the Fruit of Life. Before the trituration, three of the women provers swam naked in a pool in the stunning gorge as already mentioned above.

There was a real celebration of being in complete acceptance of our bodies - however we might individually feel about our own bodies. The other women were discreet in watching, and really celebrated the beauty of all of the bodies.

As one prover said: “We have seen each other naked, and have been able to be free - just as we are.”. Another who had swum in the pool felt there was no judgement about her body.

I prover reflected on how she had put on a bit of weight, and yet felt greater acceptance of and peace with her body.

As another prover said “I looked at every naked woman and every woman looked beautiful."

We were reminded of the work of Dr Michael Newton and his books *Journey of Souls* and *Destiny of Souls.* Michael Newton is a hypnotherapist who was only focused on material aspects of his work; helping people lose weight or stop smoking. After over one hundred clients spontaneously travelled to “life between lives” space, did he start to recognise that this was worth documenting. His clients all had similar experiences. They all described that, in the in-between moments between lifetimes, when we choose the life we are coming in to, that we also choose our bodies. The books describe that we are given a choice of three different bodies, and our soul chooses which one it would like to experience. There is no judgement at all; the invitation is simply for the soul to have an experience. There was a wondering of what might happen if we were to come to a place of acceptance around our bodies, knowing that we have chosen them, rather than making our bodies wrong in some way, or comparing ourselves based on societal or cultural pressures as to what constitutes a beautiful body.

This remedy helps us to remember that every body is beautiful. This may be a useful remedy for those who use augmentation or harsh cosmetic treatments.

Connection with Nature - especially Bees

During the tritiation, we deeply connected with ants, birds and crabs - and especially bees!

We heard and saw ravens, crows and ring necked parrots.

Ants, birds, crabs and bees live in communities. Ants came up to us on the large egg shaped rock we were sitting on to triturate. As one prover said: "The ants might be able to smell the sugar. It is interesting because they represent industry and collaboration for the greater good. We are all here to do that."

A bee came and settled on the T-shirt of one of the provers. One of the provers described how bees come from Venus. We discussed how aligned with sacred geometry they are; the Phi ratios in the hexagon of the honeycomb, the Golden Spiral dance they weave as they fly and we talked about the vision that bees have.

All of these have a significant connection with energetic resonance - some that we know of through sound, but perhaps all respond to sounds that we cannot hear as humans.

We discussed a situation where a woman who had been in considerable pain from a condition for a long time, and where nothing had worked, had been stung by 2 bees. Her pain vanished. Later, when she studied the exact location of each sting, each corresponded to an acupuncture meridian point. They just felt the resonance of what she needed energetically, and brought her healing.

One prover described her experience of sitting inside an art installation where the sound of bees wings was played, and how deeply mesmerising, and profoundly regulating of the nervous system that sound was.

Pollination also emerged as an aspect of this remedy.

We felt very connected to nature and the sacredness, beauty and peacefulness of the gorge we were in. It brought such comfort and stillness, connect and groundedness, as we have described.

Vision

There were several references to the eyes, to vision and to perception. One prover said "The colours I see seem vibrant. This is a remedy for the eyes. Vision is not just about what you see."

When we understand that this is a remedy for the feminine, for women who literally bear the fruit of life in having babies, and that babies are often visioned in a mother's mind's eye and heart before they arrive, it seems like a natural progression to appreciate the connection with vision.

There was a reminder that the eyes are the gateway to the soul, through which we can experience deep connection, especially when gazing deeply into the eyes of another. Intimacy can be said to literally mean "into me I see". Our eyes facilitate deep intimacy with another.

Cosmic & Body Cycles

This remedy connects us with important cosmic cycles, just as it does with hormonal cycles in our bodies. We discussed Venus, Jupiter and Sirius and the cycles that govern our journeys, especially the expansive cycles that were present during that time.

Circadian rhythms are our body's natural, internal 24-hour cycles that regulate sleep-wake patterns, hormones and our appetite. These are guided by light and darkness in your environment, and are controlled by a master clock in the hypothalamus - the suprachiasmatic nucleus (SCN). The Fruit of Life, with it's relationship with cycles, and endings and beginnings (akin to the move between light and dark) helps regulate the sleep and wake cycles. This is a useful remedy to consider for disrupted sleep patterns, for those who work shift patterns, and one to add to arnica for long distance air travel.

In the way that there is acceptance of the body, this remedy also brings an acceptance of time.

Mental / Emotional Symptoms

Death of a loved one
Difficulties letting go of a loved one in transition
Difficulties letting go during transition
Difficulties accepting situations in life

Needing control
Anxiety
Resistance to acceptance
Resistance to letting go
Grief
Depression
Chaos
A need for stillness
Hurried, hasty
Overthinking
Overwork
Workaholic
Too much to do
Always doing something
Busy
Lack of peace
Lack of stillness
Ungrounded
Time feels hurried
Need for peace
Many challenges - not knowing what to address first
Feeling constricted and constrained
Nothing matters
Needing to move, expanding - permission to occupy space
Feeling ugly
Shyness about body
Body dysmorphia
Need for self-acceptance
Lack of appreciation of partner
Not feeling listened to by partner
Not listening to / hearing / seeing partner
Post partum depression
Fear of impending labour (pregnant mothers)

Physical Particular Symptoms

Head

Headache from lack of regular sleep
Headache from disturbed sleep patters

Eyes

Dull vision
Blurred vision
Difficulties making eye contact

Ears

Lack of connection with the sounds of nature

Lungs & Breathing

Anxious breathing
Shallow breathing
Asthma triggered by anxiety

Heart

Heart palpitations
Stagnant flow of blood
Irregular heartbeat
Blood clots

Digestion

Constipation
Diarrhoea - watery, gushing
Diarrhoea - caused by anxiety
Foul smelling stools

Stomach

Anxiety in stomach
Knot in the stomach
Promotes flow of gastric juices

Liver

Stagnant liver
Cleanses liver
Inflammation in liver

Kidneys

Cleanses kidneys
Proteinuria
Inflammation in kidneys

Bladder

Retention of urine
Frequency of urination
Burning sensation when urinating
Forked stream of urine
Dark coloured urine
Cystitis

Female Reproductive

Irregular cycles
Dysmenorrhea
Amenorrhoea
Dark blood
Blood clots
Menarche - to establish cycles with ease
Menopause
Labour - slow progress
Labour - not letting go into the experience

Male Reproduction

Poor quality sperm
Low sperm count

Back and Limbs

Painful toes
Stiffness - better movement

Physical General Symptoms

Sleep

Poor quality sleep
Disrupted sleep
Change of time zones
Waking early with too many thoughts
Difficulty falling asleep
Restless sleep

Dreams

Dreams of travelling
Dreams of conception
Dreams of new beginnings

Body Temperature

Chilly

Food & Drink

Desire for bread
Desire for crackers
Desire for melon

Energy Levels

High energy
Restlessness

Clinical

Anaemia
Constipation
Diarrhoea
Dying
Infertility
Body dysmorphia

Spiritual

Death & transformation
Birth & transformation
Rebirth
Shedding
Letting go
Stillness and calm
Sacred feminine holding space for sacred masculine
The true reciprocal / circular reciprocal of the feminine and masculine
Lions Gate portal
Eyes as gateways to the soul
Sisterhood
Souls' journey of choosing body

Remedy Affinities

Aconite
Arg nit
Arsenicum
Ayahuasca
Buddleia
Chamomilla
Dodona
Frankincense
Green
Mastic Gum
Nettle
Oak
Purple
Sandalwood

Silver birch
Vesica Piscis

Tree of Life

13 August 2025
Lilla
Watarrka Land
Northern Territory
Australia

7 provers were involved with this trituration, all 7 were women. This was triturated using the intuitive trituration method to a 13c.

"This is a remedy of the universe."

The Tree of Life

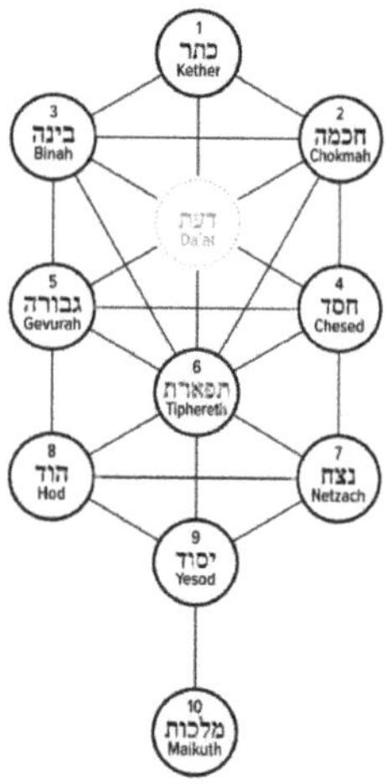

The Tree of Life is a symbol taught in the Kabbalah. It represents the journey of our soul - it is a map for our pathway to God. Each of the circles (Sephirot) corresponds to an important aspect of life that is part of the journey to Source. The Tree of Life, like all of the sacred geometry symbols sits within the Flower of Life.

There are 11 Sephirot, however usually only 10 are taught - there is an extra "hidden" one. The 10 Sephirot correspond to the 7 chakra system - and the 11th "hidden" Sephirot corresponds with the 8th chakra - the Thymus Chakra. I teach Pythagorean and Phi mathematics in how the 8 chakras form an octave, which generate - as Pythagoras taught - *harmonia.*

The ten main Sephirot are:

- Keter (closest to Source)
- Binah (understanding)
- Chochmah (wisdom)
- Gemurah (strength of boundaries)
- Chesed (loving & kindness)
- Tifaret (harmony & beauty)
- Hod (surrender)
- Netzach (victory)
- Yesod (foundation)
- Malkut (manifestation & sovereignty)

Da'at is the 11th Sephirot that can be hidden. It corresponds to knowledge. The Thymus chakra, which is associated with it, connects us with our time-line; with every lifetime we have ever lived - and the knowledge that we have gathered as a soul through time.

The left side of the Tree of Life connects with the feminine, and the right side with the masculine, so there is also a balance of the masculine and feminine found in the Tree of Life.

Tree of Life Homeopathic Remedy™

Key Themes

Spiritual Knowledge & Wisdom
Angelic Kingdom
Essenes
Transcending the Patriarchy
Interconnectedness with nature
Community
Inclusion / exclusion
Sacred Communication

Truth
Inner Journey
Healthy boundaries
Balance of Masculine & Feminine
The Mother
Sovereignty

Spiritual Knowledge & Wisdom

There was a considerable amount of discussion around spiritual knowledge and wisdom amongst the provers.

We discussed the Indigenous songlines. A songline (or Dreaming track) in Australian Indigenous culture is "a vast, ancient, spiritual map encoded in songs, stories, dance, and art, tracing the paths of creator ancestors who shaped the land, providing navigation, law, history, and crucial survival knowledge (food, water, social rules) across vast territories, acting as a "cultural passport". These melodic journeys connect sacred sites, linking people and places across generations and language groups, functioning as living libraries of ecological and social wisdom."

We reflected on the 144 disciples of Jesus, the Mayan Calendar, the Mystery Schools of Egypt and Archangel Metatron's teachings on the Divine Electron as found in the channelled book *The Keys of Enoch.*

The Divine Electron is an understanding of how the electron is not merely a subatomic particle but a "free-flowing stream of electronic light" or a "vital spark" that serves as the basis for all physical and energetic forms.

According to the *Keys of Enoch*, the universe is structured in seven densities or realms, ranging from the most ethereal to the most material, each governed by specific frequencies and laws.

We shared how in Ancient teachings, it only takes 144,000 beings that can shift the energy. This has been shown in the Maharishi experiments conducted in 1993 where research showed a direct correlation between large numbers of meditators (around 4000), meditating on peace in Washington DC and Chicago, and a proportional reduction in violent crime, using Transcendental Meditation (TM) techniques.

One prover said: "I am experiencing a direct line all the way up to the centre of the universe through milky way down through crown [chakra] and into the Earth. It is a blue light - between a pale blue and electric blue and it has a fluorescence. It is like a gateway connecting to the stars. This is where the knowledge is that we are bringing down to the Earth."

There was also a deep connection felt with the Essenes; the tribe that Jesus and Mary Magdalene and Mother Mary were all said to be from. They lived with equality between men and women and there were said to have been as many female and male disciples. The Essenes lived humble lives, and devoted their time to seeking Oneness with God, practising the highest vibrational teachings learned from the Mystery Schools in Egypt and from around the world. They knew how to directly commune with God, and did not use an intermediary (eg a Priest, Imam or Rabbi). The highest expression of a communion with God was the ability to practice "light conception"; conception born out of light - and it is said that Mother Mary was conceived by light in the body of her mother Anna, as well as Jesus. The Dead Sea Scrolls, which mainly reside in the vaults of the Vatican, are the teachings of the Essenes.

One prover shared "How extraordinary that the Dead Sea Scrolls and the Nag Hammadi Library were exposed to us within a few years [of each other]. The Dead Sea Scrolls were Old Testament and the Nag Hammadi Library is where the Gospel of Thomas comes in. There was a power grab by the Vatican. In the Nag Hammadi Library, there was knowledge of that we are souls traversing heaven again and again and the Vatican has hidden this stuff - because when the Nag Hammadi Library was first discovered, a scholar translated it before realising it is dynamite."

This is a remedy that connects us with their wisdom once more.

Angelic Kingdom

There was a deep connection with the Angelic Kingdom experienced with this proving, in particular Archangel Metatron and Archangel Michael.

The angels are said to be in Ancient teachings beings that are closest to God; that they are messengers that connect us with the pure unconditional love of Source (or God).

There are Archangels that oversee each Sephirot, acting as channels for divine energy, intelligence, and consciousness between God and humanity. In particular:

- Keter (Crown): Archangel Metatron (often seen as the highest, linking to the Crown).
- Chokmah (Wisdom): Archangel Raziel (the "Secret of God").
- Binah (Understanding): Archangel Tzafkiel (or Tzaphkiel)
- Da'at (Knowledge): Archangel Uriel
- Chesed (Mercy/Kindness): Archangel Tzadkiel (or Zadkiel).
- Gevurah (Judgment/Strength): Archangel Kamael (or Camael / Chamuel)
- Tiferet (Beauty/Harmony): Archangel Michael (often paired with Raphael).
- Netzach (Victory/Endurance): Archangel Uriel
- Hod (Glory/Splendor): Archangel Michael (sometimes paired

with Archangels Uriel or Raphael) Yesod (Foundation): Archangel Gabriel

- Malkuth (Kingdom/Manifestation): Archangel Sandalphon (connecting the spiritual to the physical).

One prover also talked about the Elohim - who are the highest geometric beings. Elohim is sometimes used as a Hebrew word for God, but it can refer to angels, humans, rulers.

This is a remedy that helps us to connect with the Angelic Realms.

Transcending the Patriarchy

There was a clear understanding that this is a remedy to help rebalance many of the effects of the patriarchy - for example a lack of sovereignty, lack of knowledge, a disconnection from wisdom, a transgression or suppression of boundaries, a loss of strength, and a distraction away from God or Source.

Interconnectedness with nature

This is a remedy that reminds us of our interconnectedness with nature. As one prover said: "I think the Tree of Life is the pathway. There is no one way - it is a personal journey. Anchored in our understanding of it is also the understanding of roots and trees, the mycelial network and how [we now know that the trees] talk and communicate and that trees look after each other. Experiments conducted in arboreal forests in North America have found that the trees look after their little ones but also other species and the eco system. The mushrooms are the brains and do the intercommunication. This is about communication, perfection one nature."

Community including ancestors

This remedy invites connection with community. Some of the provers felt they were connected in with rings of ancestors around them.

There was also a sense of lightness and laughter, community and togetherness, and a sense of support from others. As one prover shared: "There is peace....with each other, once we come back to the present, the amount of support and truth and healing that can come is wonderful. This remedy calls in support from the outside., but the type of support that comes in is so aligned and nurturing. It is a connector. One that connects."

Another prover reflected on the gifts we learned about how the Indigenous peoples sing the songs of the land. "I loved when we stopped the car and [our guide] spoke about the songs [the Indigenous people sing]. They speak the songs and words into the land. There is a geographical grid - there is a metaphysical grid - that is understood. I love how the Indigenous peoples understand the plants and they speak their healing properties, as well as the resonance and vibrations of the song lines."

It was noted that the words and songs in the song lines are passed down person to person and not written down.

Inclusion / exclusion

One prover shared grief about having experienced exclusion from a community. She had felt a sense of a lack of balance for some time.

We also talked about the divisions that mean some people are included or excluded based on what they believe - and how these divisions still occur within more conscious communities.

"We want to fear something or we want to worship it. There is still division; a sense of "I know something you don't know, and I will make fun of your beliefs" which is still division that we see in so-called "conscious communities". There is still an energy of divide and conquer that we can see - for example in the debate on viruses and whether they are real or not."

Sacred communication

One prover shared a beautiful insight into black cockatoos.

"They are an endagered species, with a maximum of 20 years left. They nest in the same tree that they were born in. They dig a hollow with their beaks, then the bird lays one egg. They live in flocks, and every member of the family has a special part to play in the the collective song, they are like an orchestra. When one member passes away, the song cannot be sung again."

It is known that many parent birds will sing to their babies, and teach them the sounds of the calls. Late-stage embryos often chip inside the shell to communicate with the mother - especially when they are ready to hatch.

The voice is really important in sacred communication. As one prover said, however: "The voice creates and a voice can destroy."

There is also the reminder here of what was explored under the Key Theme of Interconnectedness with Nature.

Truth

There was a conversation about truth. When we are aligned with ourselves, and we have a connection to this, we can draw healthy boundaries - and align with our sovereignty.

One prover said "Truth is where the mind is hence battle of the mind. If we free the mind the heart will work well to connect us with truth."

Another prover shared that "there is a balance between the mind and ego and the heart. It is all about balance - about mastery."

There was a sharing about how the Tree of Life connects us with the truth about the self. There is a meditative practice for aligning with the truth of the self using a "Self-Realization Mantra" that correlates different states of being with the sephirot of the Tree:

- Malkuth (Kingdom/Physical World): "I Am Thee Iself." (Acknowledging the individual physical self).
- Yesod (Foundation/Subconscious): "I Am Thee Allself." (Connecting to the universal field).
- Tiferet (Beauty/Harmony/Self): "I Am Thee Godself." (The heart of the tree; the higher self).
- Da'at (Knowledge/Abyss): "I Am Thee Noself." (Transcendent emptiness/ego dissolution).
- Kether (Crown/Divine Will): "I Am Thee Amness." (Pure beingness).

It was felt that this remedy strengthens these connection with the truth of the self. This in turn helps us to experience alignment in our centre.

Another prover shared: "Our inner journey; looking inwards at our own shadows, moving through the different stages of the tree, all of the journey is us looking within to all the places that are blocking us and stopping us from moving into our full capacity, noticing our shadows and shining light on all our judgements, all that we are withholding or judging, shining a light and finding out what we can let go of, what is no longer serving us, what keeps us from being our full expression. There is always another thing."

Inner Journey

This is a remedy that invites an inner journey; to connect with and reclaim the different aspects of ourselves in order to strengthen our pathway to and connection with God. As one prover said: "Your inner journey, looking inwards, own shadows, moving through the different stages of the tree, all of the journey is us looking within to all the places that are blocking us and stopping us from moving into our full capacity. Noticing our shadows and shining light on all our judgements, all that we are withholding or judging, shining a light and finding out what we can let go of, what is no longer serving us. What keeps us from being our full expression? There is always another thing to explore and transform."

Healthy boundaries

Holding healthy boundaries is an important key theme in this remedy. Whereas Carcinosin and Staphysagria can stimulate the vital force to express boundaries vehemently, this is a remedy that calls for a return to a balanced, poised, aligned, strong centre, based on a deep knowing of resonance and truth.

I was reminded of what I have learned growing up in the Serbian Orthodox Church. "The importance of healthy boundaries has been written out of many religions, and replaced with a sense of service that requires putting others' needs first. In the Christian Orthodox Church, candles are lit to hour each of our loved ones - one candle for each person we would like to be lit by God. We always light candles for the living before we light candles for the dead, as the message is that we must always think of the living first, and before lighting any candles for anyone else, we always light a candle for ourselves first. We kiss the candle, thinking of ourselves or our loved one - whoever the candle is for - and then cross ourselves and light. Honouring ourselves first is important - there is an understanding that we cannot look after others unless we look after and love ourselves first." Another prover added "Orthodoxy first started the break away in 325CE at the Council of Nicaea - until then the soul was seen as eternal and they needed to write that out so the Orthodox split off. It is a much more real religion." [Orthodoxy and Catholicism finally fully split in what is known as *The Great Schism* in 1054AD].

As we discussed this, one prover noticed that she was really studying Orion's Belt in the night sky. It is an interesting reflection that we learned about the Dreamtime story of the Pleiades as told by the Indigenous Australians, which I will share more about in the proving of The Pleiades. A short summary is that Orion has a trickster, lustful energy and chases the Seven Sisters (Pleiades) across the sky. His trickster energy causes two of the Seven Sisters to become excluded, and their journey is harder although more rewarding in the end.

It is interesting, on reflection and understanding the significance of the Dreamtime story of the Pleiades, that the prover was looking up at Orion whilst we were discussing the Great Schism.

Two provers left early during this trituration; honouring their boundaries and need for rest (leaving five provers, like in the story of the Pleiades, that we didn't know about at the time of the trituration!).

One prover had draw a card just before coming to the proving. She said: "There is a picture of the hearth fire and people sitting around, show me this journey and its that picture, it is about fellowship, hearth fire, joining with family, in the interest of pursuing common pursuits. It is all about fellowship.". Another prover shared that: "The gathering of friends around emotional intelligence, and safety is a powerful experience, these are bonding experiences, growing with comrades, with family or friends."

Another prover was reflecting on the responses of community after a loved one has passed. "People are so caring. Some say odd things....however we do not have to be alone, we can feel there is a difference between being alone and lonely. People are fundamentally kind."

Another prover sensed the "support, not automatically from outside, more the foundations are solid, so we can feel that they are there."

The healthy boundaries are also established by focusing on what matters, and coming back to simplicity: "It is really simple, It is simply that, reminded today that we were driven through such a beautiful landscape, remember with this remedy to walk with the trees."

Balance of Masculine & Feminine

The provers discussed at length the exclusion of women from society and life, particularly in relation to the example of the Essenes and the balance that they lived with.

This is a remedy that restores a balance of masculine and feminine.

The Mother

One prover talked about Asherah (also known as Ishtar), saying "she was known as Queen of Heaven, Mother of Creation. She represented Divine Wisdom and the Tree of Life. King Josiah in 623 BC removed from the Temple the symbol of the goddess Asherah, burnt it, pounded its ashes to dust, and scattered it over the public burial ground. She was written out of all of the historical texts and demoted to Eve, and made the fallen. This was the start of the patriarchy and the demotion of women."

Dr Deanna Riddick describes how "she is considered the matriarch (Creatress) and El was the Patriarch (Creator). She was the female consort to the Hebrew God Yahweh and was widely worshiped by Israelites, Canaanites and many others."

We were reminded of how the Essenes honoured women and the sacredness of the Mother.

One prover was reading *The Witch Trials* at the time of this trip, and felt it was particularly relevant to this proving.

There was also a discussion about the encapsulating of the placenta and stem cells after birth. As one prover said: "The placenta looks like the one world tree. It connects the baby to the mother and to the cosmos - a ladder into the uterus."

Sovereignty

The provers discussed the rise of people being in their sovereignty and how more people waking up to the structures of the world around them. This is particularly reflected in the rise of homeschooling, as was discussed by the provers.

One prover received a text message from a friend that said: "Today 13th is the day of highest manifestation of the lions gate (8/8) - the symbol off divine feminine. Align and step into trusting your soul destiny. Be bold, and unapologetic."

Mental / Emotional Symptoms

Feeling disconnected from God / a Higher Power / Source
Disconnected from nature
Feeling of disconnection from communities / purpose / self / loved ones
Difficulties communicating or expressing needs, wishes and desires
Poor boundaries
Imbalance in masculine / feminine
Feeling motherless
Sovereignty
Unresolved karma
Difficulties identifying truth
Difficulties making decisions
Lack of trust in oneself
Lack of self-belief
Karma = unresolved energy.
Lack of balance - too much in the head or too much in the heart
Grief from exclusion / excommunication
Lack of alignment
Feeling powerless
Feeling helpless
Needing more solid foundations
Not living full potential
Unhappiness
Addictions
Balanced empowerment in men
Balanced empowerment in women

Physical Particular Symptoms

Head

Pain in occiput
Headache from overthinking
Pain on left side of forehead
Dandruff (seborrhoeic)

Eyes

Pain in left eye

Ears

Muffled hearing
Blocked ears (earwax)

Nose

Snoring

Throat

Stuttering
Difficulties expressing oneself

Lungs & Breathing

Anxious, shallow breathing

Heart

Impaired heart valves

Digestion

Leaky gut
Microbiome imbalance
Inflammation

Stomach

Acid indigestion / reflux

Liver

Sluggish liver
Detoxification

Female Reproductive

Placental insufficiency
Painful periods
Low libido
Excess libido

Male Reproduction

Impotence
Low libido
Excess libido

Back & Limbs

Pain in right shoulder hurting, feel really heavy, need to stretch
Lumbar tension
Tightness and soreness on the right trapezius muscle.

Sleep

Insomnia
Poor sleep
Early waking

Dreams

Dreams of travelling to distant lands
Dreams of travelling back in time
Dreams of angels
Spiritual dreams.

Energy Levels

Feeling heavy, lumbar tension
Very tired
Suddenly tired
Need for sleep and rest

Spiritual

Patriarchy and demotion of the feminine
Voice as creative and destructive
Thymus chakra, 8th chakra, Pythagoras
Connection to divine electron
Connection with Angelic Kingdom including Archangels Metatron and Michael
144,000 beings can shift energy
Mystery schools, keys of Enoch, Mayan calendar, the Essenes
Healing, balance, and mastery
Rings of ancestors, love prevailing
Personal sovereignty and boundaries
Orthodox candle ritual and soul eternity
Mary Magdalene and sacred apostles

Orion's Belt symbolism
Songlines and land connection
Dead Sea Scrolls and Nag Hammadi Library, Vatican suppression
Angelic orders and anchoring divine connection
Mushroom/mycelium communication networks
Past life visions, connection to Jesus, Isis, and ancient medicine
Truth, division, awakening
Personal spiritual journeys, inner shadows, and release
Fellowship, community, and shared journeys.

Clinical

Remedy Affinities

Ambra grisea
Arg nit
Buddleja
Butterfly
Carcinosin
Chelidonium
Emerald
Gelsemium
Graphites
Kali phos
Lycopodium
Oak
Olive Tree
Petrified Sequoia
Psorinum
Pulsatilla
Red
Tarentula
Silica
Silver birch
Staphysagria

Grid of Life

16 August 2025
Yulara
Northern Territory
Australia

11 provers were involved with this trituration, 10 were women, and 1 was a man. This was triturated using the intuitive trituration method to a 12c. We were joined by Michal Yakir, Sarah Valentini, Paul Degonda & Cara Munn for this trituration.

The day of this trituration we had visited Kata-Tjuta, an incredible rock formation near Uluru. Where Uluru expresses a more feminine energy, Kata-Tjuta connected with a more masculine energy. We very much walked and connected with Kata-Tjuta in a silent reverence. We had usually been a chatty group, but silence felt important in his presence.

The Grid of Life

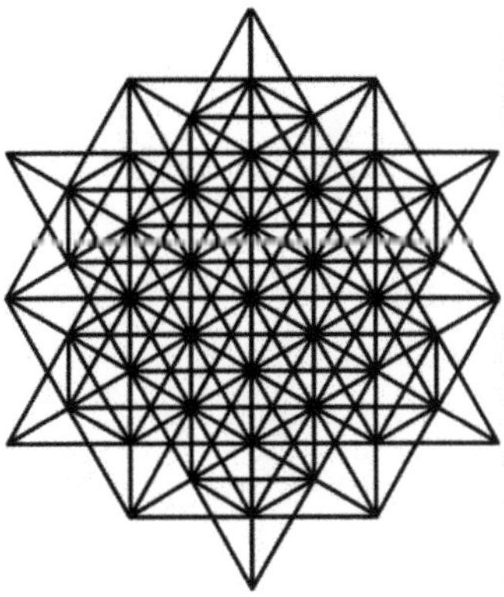

The Grid of Life is a grid of 64 tetrahedrons.

The number 64 is hugely important in the natural world - there are 64 codons in human DNA, 64 is the number of cells we have before they start to differentiate after conception, there were 64 manifestations of Lord Shiva, 64 hexagrams in the I Ching.

Within the Grid of Life is also formed a Vector Equlibrium, which you can read about in the later proving - however for now in essence it represents the moving from polarity to unity; from duality to centre, stillness and balance.

The Grid of Life symbolises linking our own individual path in harmony with our soul / star family. Doing so we can then amplify the energy available to accomplish and manifest (or materialise) our goals - and really show up in service to something much bigger.

Grid of Life Homeopathic Remedy™

Key Themes

Communication, Truth & Misunderstandings
Connection
Over-apologising
Cracks, Breaks and Healing
Spiritual and Multidimensional Experiences
Interconnectedness with the animal kingdom, ancestors, star & soul family
Alignment in relationships
Mother Energy

Communication, Truth & Misunderstandings

One prover drew a divination card - it was all about the throat chakra. The message was one that said: "This card symbolises your connection to self expression through speech. This is about your ability to speak your truth, which comes naturally to you, but it's not always well received by listeners. This struggle to speak your mind has often landed you in hot water, and created unwanted attention. These experiences have left you cautious to speak out and be heard. Your fears of persecution for speaking your truth are well founded and are related to other lifetimes where you have been punished for not surrendering to general consensus. These times are different and now you have to practice upsetting the status quo if you're to be true to yourself. A massive weight will be lifted from you when you finally acknowledge what has been keeping you awake at night. Find the voice from within and own your truth. No more internal conversations, the time to talk is now or you will miss an amazing opportunity where people will gladly listen to what you have to say. As long as you are speaking what you believe, then it is your truth. It may not be what others believe, however it is your reality and on this occasion it will be shared by many who don't have the courage to speak out to themselves."

What became interesting at this point was that our guests felt tired, and left, as it was late in the evening.

After this, we discussed the experience, which was a beautiful one, with our guests. However each of us had a completely different perception of one part of the evening! This felt completely relevant to the proving of this remedy.

One prover said: "The first thing we do as women is assume we are doing things wrong and to hold a burden that is not there. As women a lot is self-imposed, there are so many layers to all the perceptions. It is really about each person's truth and taking ownership - this is mine, this is not mine." This prover went on to so eloquently say: "There are so many truths." In our misperceptions, we create a "self-imposed suffering....we create our own suffering."

One prover talked about the story of Henry Vth, which Shakespeare turned into a play because of how Shakespearean the story is. "I didn't know the story of Henry the 5th until I watched the film *The King* on Netflix. And wow. It is the story of how every war begins. Henry Vth went to war with France, but only because his advisors kept feeding a narrative that the son of the King of France was sending him insults. At first Henry Vth ignored all these messages, because he didn't want war - he was a reluctant king. But his advisors kept giving him messages about what the French King's son was allegedly doing, and kept poking until Henry Vth wages war on France. Eventually Henry Vth works out that it was all set up - that war was waged to unite the common folk behind the King. The same has happened again and again through history."

Wars (and any disagreements) being fed by manipulation, lies, people spreading mistruths about others. So much division happens because of this behaviour.

As one prover said: "In hunter-gatherer times - no one was more important - if you were the shaman, it was because you were good at being the shaman. The chief was good at being the chief. When there was a discussion, everyone spoke their truth, passing the stick, that is enough, everyone had been heard and spoke their truth, it was a considered approach."

I am reminded of how a technique of the patriarchy is to divide and conquer, for people to take others aside and whisper in their ears about others. Indigenous tribes apply the wisdom of sitting together. We are less likely to say things that are demeaning about others in front of the person we are talking about, because there is no room for shadow to emerge. It is in the shadow that mistruths and miscommunication occur.

We were reminded of Don Miguel Ruiz's Four Agreements[41]:

1. Be Impeccable with Your Word - Speak with integrity, use words to uplift, not harm.
2. Don't Take Anything Personally - Others' actions reflect their own reality, not yours.
3. Don't Make Assumptions - Ask questions to avoid misunderstandings
4. Always Do Your Best - Our best varies day to day, but to try our

41 https://www.thefouragreements.com/

best in that moment.

Connection

We explored compassion and acceptance and the importance of listening, holding space, and creating safe environments for expression and connection.

One prover shared an example of a time she was managing a long-standing member of staff who was perceived to be difficult. "I just sat and listened to her. She had been ignored for years, and I just felt like she needed to be heard. So I had a meeting with her, and she talked about all the things that bothered her. I just listened and then when the meeting came to an end, I told her I couldn't necessarily fix things, but that I had heard her that was all she needed. After that, she worked well, without complaint, and smiled at me every time I walked past her. Sometimes that's all we need, is to be heard without judgement and then we can move on."

Everyone's truth is different. As one prover said: "We are all interconnected and one. I am being reminded of when looking at another we are seeing a reflection of ourselves, we are seeing an unhealed part sometimes, but always a reflection, holding out mirrors for ourselves."

This remedy celebrates the process of bonding, inclusion, and returning to unity after separation or conflict.

Even though there was a seriousness in this proving, we also were able to deeply reflect - and laugh at ourselves too. As one prover said: "It's important we carry it lightly".

One prover shared the story of a rave story that is coming to Netflix - about a woman who hadn't been a raver, but when her husband died, she found rave music as a healing journey for her grief. We reflected on the lies that had been told about ecstasy and the rave movement, when actually it was a movement that was about deep and profound connection.

One prover then sounded the crystal bowl, and talked about how she could see the sound waves emanating from the bowl for about 30 seconds. Another prover continued the conversation about sound in raves: "back in the 90s, you would dance on or next to speakers that were the size of doors. You could see the sound vibrations booming out of the speakers, you could feel the vibrations pulsating through your body. Raves brought people together for one single purpose, and that purpose was to experience one love."

We finished the proving with a lot of lightness and laughter. As one prover described it: "The kind of laughter where one person teeny smirks and another starts laughing - they set each other off......the laughter of people who are truly connected."

Over-apologising

One prover commented: "I keep hearing people apologising all the time - it feels like not wanting to take up space in the world. I have to apologise for being myself, I hear women apologising all the time. I feel like women epigenetically had no power for thousands of years, anything we did could be used....we couldn't own land, we were powerless, there is fear in our epigenetics. We are overly apologising thinking we are bring courteous, when we are actually keeping ourselves small.

We talked about how there are cultures in the world where people generally don't apologise as much - not from a place of being rude, but from a place of accepting that each person is just expressing themselves.

Cracks, Breaks and Healing

Before each remedy was made during the trip to the Northern Territory in Australia, a beautiful large crystal bowl aligned with the Crown Chakra was played. On this occasion two of the provers could see the sound waves around the bowl vibrating. One heard the sound waves travelling differently to each ear, being played separately before sounding as one.

One prover said: "I am confused, nothing makes sense, I feel anger and fright. Before that I saw a big crack, but it is something you see between continents, greyish, separating continents in the shape of a snake. There is a big mark of snakes on the rocks, discussed at the centre today....also there is a big crack in the land. One was my personal feeling and the other was my personal vision."

Another prover shared: "There is a feeling of fear, as though there is a big event, but also this is life. I was just watching it from afar. That's what happened - there was a crack and a break." Other provers shared they were experiencing or hearing cracks in their knees.

One prover said: "This is a remedy for healing the cracks".

Another prover highlighted that "Reptilian nature is - we are in constant threat - and that keeps people in opposition."

We were then told one of the Indigenous stories of cracks in the land. Each tribe and each language has it's own version of these stories, so this is but one: "A powerful female ancestor who was a snake became enraged after her nephew was killed, and her grief and anger drove her to seek justice. A woman's love for her family is so huge that she is willing to protect them - so with the story, when Indigenous people do something wrong they get a punishment. Acting under traditional law, she strikes the snake responsible for the death, hitting him across the head several times. These blows leave two cracks on his body, which are visible in the landscape today. The cracks are not just physical marks but permanent reminders of what occurred and of the consequences of breaking the law.."

We were also reminded of the Japanese art of Kintsugi - filling cracks with gold. The repair becomes part of the object's beauty, embracing imperfection, and often making the restored item more precious.

Following on from this, we connected with a different type of crack - the opening of the fabric of reality that the *Subtle Knife* in Philip Pullman's book is able to do, that enables characters to move between dimensions and worlds.

Spiritual and Multidimensional Experiences

One prover felt that she was using telekinesis. She said: "I have this sense of telekinesis - the way the wood is shifting, I just have this sense that I am doing it with my eyes. There is a sense of control."

We explored UFOs and travel through time and space - the connection with the stars that is so inherent in the spiritual significance of the Grid of Life.

Interconnectedness with the natural world, animal kingdom, ancestors, star & soul family

Several provers experienced curiosity from the animal kingdom. One said: "I saw a reptile move in closer, a claw closely, it was not scary, but a guardian energy, was not fearful, curious. I have never seen the reptiles move in like that before, feels like there is a lot of wisdom, the animal kin are moving closer towards us." Another said:

"It feels like claws are massaging my feet. I am picturing a dragon foot." It turned out that this was a perentie lizard - they are black with yellow spots and can grow up to 2m in length.

We talked about the Komodo Dragon proving led by homeopath Kate Birch.

We could also hear dingos howling outside - both the reptiles and the dingos are, as one prover highlighted, ancient DNA animals.

As one prover said, "there is a feeling of the animal kin moving in", to which another replied "out here the ancestors are animals so they shape shift."

It feels important to point out here that ancestors of the land will also be connected with the stars. So there is a connection between the original DNA, the animals the ancestors, and the stars. The Grid of Life connect us with the stars, and with our original soul and star family.

We were told of how, in Indigenous culture, ancestors shape-shift into animals.

One prover commented that it felt like we are "reactivating our original DNA".
We were reminded of relationship between reptiles and dragons, and one prover mentioned dragons forming parts of the cracks in the land in Wales.

We talked about fairies and also dinosaurs - said by some to have been dragons - and the proving of T-Rex that Danica and the Golden Spiral Proving Collective carried out. Central Australia has lots of dinosaur markings, we were told.

We also celebrated the mycelial networks, and the heart energy they bring us.

"This is a remedy that brings all the realms together", said one prover. "It calls in soul family, star family, animal and ancestral guides......that support us in our work on the Earth."

Alignment in relationships

This is a remedy that can welcome more soul and star family into our lives, and guides, however it will also gently remove those who aren't in alignment with a person's soul journey.

In this way, it has a protective element to it; like the ancestors who appeared as animals.

Mother Energy

One of the provers was 36-37 weeks pregnant during the adventure in the Northern Territory. We were really feeling the mother energy during this proving. One prover said: "I am feeling very connected to [pregnant Mama to be] - mindful of checking she is okay - is there anything we can get her. We got pillows for the Mama.

Other provers notices and celebrated the mother energy.

"Caring for the mother is caring for the child. This is love, this ability to love, it ....creates something new,."

Mental & Emotional Symptoms

Feeling confused
Nothing makes sense
Anger
Fright
Loneliness
Abandonment
Exclusion
Lack of compassion
Misunderstandings
Misperceptions
Miscommunication
Assumptions that self or other is wrong
Easily triggered by others
Brings compassion
Judgement of self or others - brings peace
Care for others
Needing to be cared for by others
Over-apologising (especially women)
Women making themselves small
Divisions - heals cracks
Need for togetherness, bonding
Welcomes support, and lightness, humour, laughter and joy
Need for connection
Pessimism
Seeing the worst in others
Fear of saying the wrong thing - and so not speaking

Physical Particular Symptoms

Head

Crack in the head
Heavy head - too many thoughts

Eyes

Blurred vision
Dullness of colours - vision
Astigmatism
Difficulties focusing on an object
Redness in sclera
Dry eyes

Ears

Hearing the same sound differently in each ear
Welcomes the sound of laughter
Tinnitus

Nose

Lachrymation - acrid, burning
Congestion - one nostril only

Mouth & Teeth

Misaligned teeth - won't repair but may call what is needed
Cavities

Throat

Difficulties speaking truth
Difficulties communicating clearly
Fear of saying the wrong thing
Tonsilitis - red sore

Lungs & Breathing

Pollution in lungs
Smoke inhalation

Heart

Athersclerosis

Digestion

Plaques / build up in colon
Dysbiosis
Leaky gut

Liver

Stones
Blockages

Kidneys

Uric acid
Kidney stones

Bladder

Cutting pains during urination
Stinging during urination

Female Reproductive

Mother-child bonding
Fertility
Blocked fallopian tubes

Male Reproduction

Sperm motility

Back & Limbs

Crack in left knee
Cracking knees

Physical General Symptoms

Sleep

Snoring

Dreams

Dreams of soul family
Dreams of star origins / family

Body Temperature

Chilly
Heat egg

Food & Drink

Energy Levels

Energy better outside
Energy better dancing, movement

Spiritual

Opens connection to star origins

Telekinesis, controlling objects with eyes
Brings in light
Opens the heart to love
Animal kin as ancestral spirits and guardians
Vision of cracks in land linked to serpent/dragon creation, multi-dimensional portal
Shape-shifting ancestors, Indigenous spiritual connection to stars and earth
Connection to mycelium as a metaphor for interconnection
Healing the cracks as a spiritual remedy
References to Uluru, rainbow serpent, ancient creation myths
Connection to multiple realms—serpents, fairies, ancestors.
Opening fabric of reality, gateways between dimensions (cracks)
Dingoes representing instinct, survival, tribal bonds
UFOs, different dimensions, cracks as portals rather than damage
Ancient people and dinosaur references linked to spiritual and physical timelines
Laughter as spiritual connection and true bonding.

Remedy Affinities

Ambra grisea
Ayahuasca
Birdsong
Blue
Causticum
Dodecahedron
Emerald
Flower of Life
Ignatia
Lac humanum
Lycopodium
Mercurius solubilis / vivus

Nat Mur
Oxytocin
Rainbow
Sea salt
Thuja
Vesica Piscis

Merkabah

16 August 2025
Yulara
Northern Territory
Australia

21 December 2025
Winter Solstice

7 provers were involved with the original trituration, all were women. This was triturated using the intuitive trituration method to a 4c. There was a further proving on 21 December 2025 with 2 provers.

The day of this trituration we had visited Kata-Tjuta, an incredible rock formation near Uluru. Where Uluru expresses a more feminine energy, Kata-Tjuta connected with a more masculine energy. We very much walked and connected with Kata-Tjuta in a silent reverence. We had usually been a chatty group, but silence felt important in his presence.

Merkabah

The Merkabah is known as the "chariot" in Hebrew. It is made of two tetrahedrons that intersect & rotate in opposite directions, which creates an energy field known as the light body (Torus) once spinning.

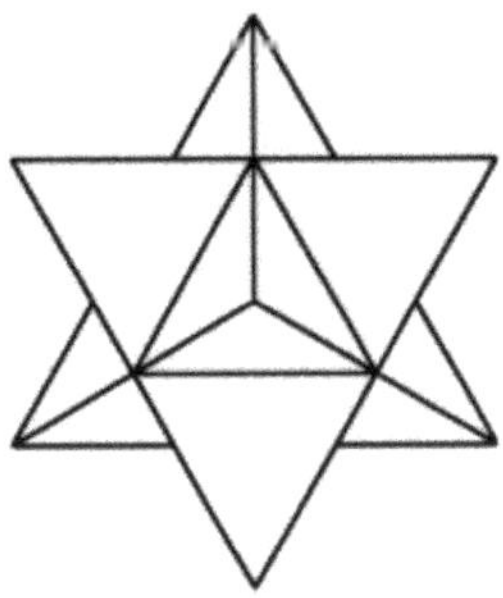

It is said that connecting with one's Merkabah can provide powerful protection, enabling us to access higher consciousness. In Chassidic Judaism, the Merkabah aligns us with all of the aspects of life, the natural world, and the Earth too. 1. Unity and Integration.

Merkabah Homeopathic Remedy™

Key Themes

Unity & Integration
Ancient Wisdom & Magic
Calm, Peace & Relaxation
Vibration (including colour and sound)
Light & Happiness

Unity & Integration

We had spent the morning at the remarkable Kata-Tjuta rock formation. We had walked in silence, and had very much gone into our own spaces. Once we returned, we had all gone off on our own, checking messages and just being on our mobile phones.

As soon as we began triturating this remedy, we felt we were easily coming together as a group once more.

On the playlist as we started the trituration was Arwen's song from Lord of the Rings.

One prover reflected upon the "Balance, harmony and integration - the spinning of the masculine and feminine tetrahedrons that enables both to flourish so there is an incredible sense of balance and connection. I can feel the new ancestors [of Yulara] and older ancestors [of a different location, Alice Springs, who had first joined us when we began our pilgrimage in the Northern Territory] standing next to each other."

Another prover noted that "this remedy is at the still point, in the middle and clicking into place, everything sorting itself out." Another said "Nothing can disturb my peace."

We discussed the balance between Mother energy - Mother Earth & Father Sky. As we did so, a Mynah bird entered the room. The name "Mynah" comes from Sanskrit, meaning "delightful" or "bubbling with joy," making it a symbol of happiness and zest for life.[42] The Mynah bird symbolizes joy, communication, adaptability, and good fortune, and are seen because of their "babbling" gift, as Divine Messengers.

Whilst we were triturating, Michal Yakir and Sarah Valentini who were also in Uluru came in to the room. It felt like unity had come in, as one prover observed: "Let's share this together"; as another said "a levelling out."

Ancient Wisdom & Magic

We talked about the Lord of the Rings, Buddha and Merlin, King Arthur and Elves, the Essenes and the fairy magic and Ancient Trees of Cornwall.

A divination card was drawn by one prover and it was the Ancient Knowledge card. It said:

"Deep within each of us is a sacred place where our most ancient knowledge is kept. These are the secrets of the past which silently await a rebirth to eagerly sent fourth knowledge which has been forgotten.

The ancient knowledge of many lifetimes laid dormant within the deepest recesses of our past and present memories. We leave such

42 https://medium.com/@absterix/winging-it-together-unraveling-life-lessons-in-myna-superstition-3cd82d5e2352

wisdom untapped for fear of what our responsibilities may be to ourselves and others if we possessed such great knowledge.

We need to allow ourselves to trust our wisdom and see searching for evidence to back up our thoughts and feelings. It's easier to look to others for the answers than to trust ourselves. We each possessed knowledge of this unique, as no one else can walk in your shoes and know your stories.

Everything we need know can be found within, and it's time to find trust in yourself and your own wisdom. It won't be long now. Your wisdom was never lost, just buried under piles of self-doubt. Self trust will soon rebirth, and you will remember what it is like to have the courage to stand in your own power and make your own decisions.[43]

One prover shared "This is about coming back to the truth, the science element - spin together, feeling the love, joy and receiving it. I want to cradle the pestle and mortar like a baby."

Another reflected on the magic: "I don't feel connected to anything artificial. It felt very artificial [when we got back] - everybody on their phone. I just want to go back to the place that feels magic, magic everywhere....I am ready to go back to magic."

One prover talked about Marko Pogačnik - a Slovenian artist and author who is fascinated by elemental beings and nature spirits.

Angels were experienced by another prover. "I feel this angelic vibration - it is light. Easeful. Supportive. This remedy is angelic."

---

43 https://solsticeshop.co.uk/products/aboriginal-goddess-chakra-oracle-by-mel-brown?srsltid=AfmBOoo845vKrX0P7bPshYYl3PnOx-OezK2ZN8b1H77iEH_wlnV9KRcA

Calm, Peace & Relaxation

We experienced a profound calmness in the room, and a lightness. One prover noticed a hopefulness in the room.

One prover shared that it "feels like transparency. The veil has been lifted through connection. There is clarity and lightness."

There was a deep feeling of relaxation in the room. Several provers slept, one later said "like an enchanted sleep", another reported feeling sleepy, gentle and peaceful.

With the deep state of relaxation and integration was the "ability to receive", .

One prover who was sleeping during the trituration dreamt of poppy fields where people wanted to sleep.

Another dreamt that she was falling off a cliff, happy to go off the cliff, no hesitation, no fear - as though she were a bird".

"Peace is a key theme here" said a prover in the second proving. "This is a remedy that dissolves all that is not light and connects us with peace."

Vibration (including colour and sound)

We were really aware of sound vibrations - including beautiful gentle music, and the sounds of the birds.

Michal talked about the evolution of plants and how the evolutionary structure is one that we cannot see with our 2D eyes as it is a 3D structure that resonates with an octave frequency. Michal talked about the fractal geometric nature of plants speaking the land (I was really seeing the Golden Spiral at this point). Michal gave us the sacred geometry view of evolution through plants

I was experiencing Michal as a beautiful elemental - faery-like - vibration. Some people immediately fell asleep when she came in.

One prover noticed how was seeing all the colours around her - she was seeing rainbow colours.

In a further proving experience, a prover noted that: "I can see all the colours of the rainbow and more. The emanating, radiating throughout my whole energy field. The colours are Dancing, Moving, flowing through all of me. I can see some pastel metallic shades of colours we would know, as well as lighter versions of the brightest colours we can see. This remedy has all the colours in it. Activates all vibrations. I feel the colours spinning around me and I feel light and happy."

Light & Happiness

This is a remedy that brings so much light and happiness. "I feel impervious to anything and everything that is not truly happy. It is a calm happiness - a contentment - rather than a jumping for joy kind of happiness. Although I am sure I could do that too. A lightness, an ease, a peaceful happiness is how I would describe it. I just feel HAPPY. At one. Happy.....It's like this remedy clears self-doubt, stills those limiting voices. It's like they feel distant and far away. I feel like I am in a meadow on a warm summer's day, and any of those voices feel like they are on a faint wind a long way away so I can barely hear them. They don't matter anymore. I am here, happy in the warm sun with wildflowers around me as I sink into a balmy, peaceful, sleepy afternoon. Everything just feels alright."

Another prover said: "I feel hope for the future".

Mental / Emotional Symptoms

Separated from others
Fragmentation
Hopelessness
Tension
Anxiety
Too busy
Life feeling out of balance
Difficulties finding time to relax
No time to rest
Intensity in life
Addictions
Too much thinking in the head
Feels weight of responsibilities

Head

Difficulties concentrating

Eyes

Cloudy vision
Blurred vision
Dull colours
Dry eyes
Itchy eyes - particularly left eye

Ears

Sensitive hearing
Blockage
Itch inside ear
Excessive wax

Nose

Congestion

Mouth & Teeth

Cavities
Decay

Throat

Sensation of tiny sharp needles in throat

Lungs & Breathing

Congestion in lungs
Clear sputum
Dry tickly cough, worse in inhalation of cold air

Digestion

Coeliac disease
Crohn's Disease

Stomach

Acid indigestion

Liver

Sluggish liver

Female Reproductive

Fertility
Sluggish energy in reproductive system - awakens energy
Hormonal imbalances

Male Reproduction

Fertility
Sluggish energy in reproductive system - awakens energy

Skin

Acne - red, sore pimples

Physical General Symptoms

Sleep

Insomnia
Difficulties falling asleep
Frequent waking - light sleep
Difficulties falling into a deep sleep
Sleep apnoea
Waking feeling unrefreshed
Interrupted sleep

Dreams

Dream of falling off a cliff, happy to go off, no hesitation, no fear - bird energy
Flying
Poppy fields

Body Temperature

Chilly

Food & Drink

Desire for green foods - salads
Desire for fresh fruit
Fats agg
Rich foods agg

Energy Levels

Sleepiness
Tiredness
Fatigue

Clinical

Coeliac disease
Crohn's disease
Constipation
Oedema
Sluggish lymph

Spiritual

Elves, King Arthur, ancient magic, Cornwall connection
Support from ancestors
Sacred geometry and fractal nature of plants
Balance/harmony and integration
Magic being cultivated and revered

Mother and father energies balance
Love

Remedy Affinities

Ayahuasca
Flower of Life
Golden Spiral
Lotus
Metatron's Cube
Milky Way
Olive
Purple
Rainbow
Silver birch
Tyrannosaurus rex

Torus

15 August 2025
Yulara
Uluru
Northern Territory
Australia

8 provers were involved with the original trituration, all were women. This was triturated using the intuitive trituration method to a 6c.

Torus

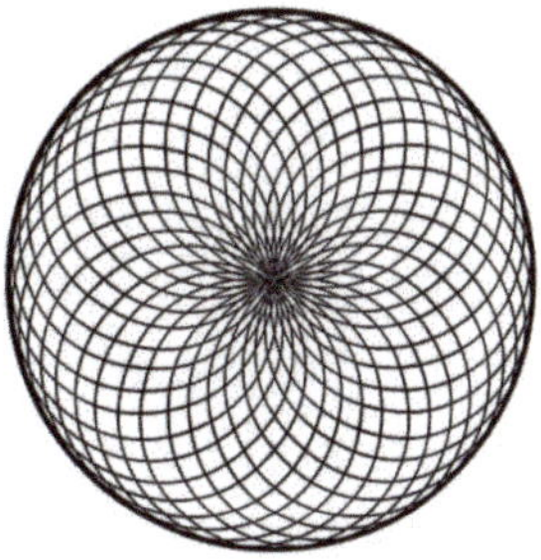

The Torus - or Toroidal Field - is a type of vortex. It is what our aura, or energetic - electromagnetic - field looks like when it is healthy, balanced and in full integrity. Our toroidal field is geometric in nature - and so built upon Phi mathematics (1.618 - the vibration of love, as Manfred Clynes discovered). Regular exposure to that which is not love can lead to a loss of the integrity of the field - we can literally develop holes in our aura. When our aura isn't strong, we can feel more sensitive, or more emotionally challenged. A loss of connection to the vibration of love can lead to trauma responses such as a lack of empathy, and behaviours that cause harm to others.

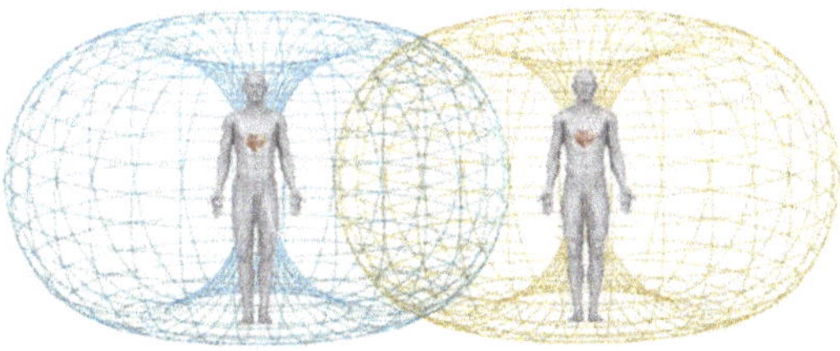

The HeartMath Institute in California has found that "The heart is the most powerful source of electromagnetic energy in the human body, producing the largest rhythmic electromagnetic field of any of the body's organs. The heart's electrical field is about 60 times greater in amplitude than the electrical activity generated by the brain. This field, measured in the form of an electrocardiogram (ECG), can be detected anywhere on the surface of the body. Furthermore, the magnetic field produced by the heart is more than 100 times greater in strength than the field generated by the brain and can be detected up to 3 feet away from the body, in all directions, using SQUID-based magnetometers".[44]

The HeartMath Institute has also performed several studies that show the magnetic signals generated by the heart have the capacity to affect individuals around us.

In 2008, Nicholas Christakis, a sociologist at Harvard University, and James Fowler, a political scientist at University of California, published a study that demonstrated that "happiness spreads among people up to three degrees of separation. That means when you feel happy, your friend's friend's friend has a higher likelihood of feeling happy too. And, it applies in both real and virtual worlds.[45] They also found that sadness spreads too, but not quite as far - not quite to three degrees.

Could it be that the way that we are spreading happiness (and sadness) is through our electromagnetic field? Could it be that an intact, whole, vital electromagnetic field is what is felt and experienced through these degrees of influence? And likewise, that a compromised electromagnetic field - torus - that has lost its wholeness and integrity also is something we can feel and

44 https://www.heartmath.org/research/science-of-the-heart/energetic-communication/#:~:text=The heart is the most,any of the body's organs.

45 https://positivepsychologynews.com/news/timothy-so/200911185246#:~:text=The research shows that within,to three degrees of separation

experience?

Because happiness spreads further than sadness, it means that the more of us that are connecting with it, and an intact toroidal field, the more change we can help naturally bring to those experiencing sadness - literally lights shining in the darkness. Bringing the electromagnetic field to a point of being intact helps everyone around us.

I am reminded of an amazing experiment conducted by brilliant Veda Austin.

She used her crystallography technique to demonstrate how the vibration of a free range egg was able to influence and transform the vibration of battery farmed eggs that surrounded it.

Literally we can be the healing light in the darkness, when we ourselves are in our light.

This, by the way, is not about bypassing. It's about transforming through the shadow into light, honouring shadow, loving shadow, not judging it, or avoiding it, but loving it.

Joseph Campbell (1904-1987). Professor of English Literature at Sarah Lawrence University in New York developed the Hero's Journey having studied the stories of all major religions and mythologies. He found that every Hero (and Heroine) faces a time when they need to "slay their dragons" - and actually, in the end, it isn't that the dragons need slaying. It is that the dragons need *loving.* That is when the Hero or Heroine is truly free. This is so beautifully depicted in the story of Luke Skywalker and Darth Vader in *Star Wars.* Luke goes back to save his Dad.

This is a remedy that welcomes the transformation from shadow into light.

It was an interesting proving to be a part of - we were really shown a tiny iota of the darkness that this remedy is here to heal. We were gifted a profound teaching, insight and learning. An energy arrived and very clearly made itself known to show us what fear can feel like. We have experienced the energy shifting to peace, gratitude and love.

Like Golden Spiral, Flower of Life, Vector Equilibrium, and Metatron's Cube, I really feel this is a remedy that benefits everyone as a support for the soul.

Torus Homeopathic Remedy™

Key Themes

Fragmentation & Division
Manipulation and Dark Forces
Struggle between Light and Darkness
Corporate Greed
Lack of Empathy
Disconnection to Connection
Healing
Protection

Fragmentation & Division

There was a strong sense of of the group splitting from the beginning - people being pulled in different directions. There was a lack of cohesiveness, and disintegration of the unity that had up until that point been very much felt in the group.
Several provers from the start described feeling annoyed. There was a reluctance to be part of the proving. Once prover said: It is the first time I feel tired and thought "I won't do this one, I will stay out of it"."
It was also noticed that:

"We are not all here together. All the other [provings] we started together."
"Division"
"Lack of cohesiveness"
"Disintegration"
"Tech has come back in and everyone is on their phones"
"Different agendas"
"Conflicting agendas"
"Everyone feels far apart - not close to each other, not close enough. I feel angry, frustrated, like I want to rage."

Manipulation and Dark Forces

One prover noticed that: "Outside forces are coming in and are pulling people in different directions. There are undercurrents."

We very much felt an energy that was demonstrating to us what darkness feels like. We felt a heaviness and darkness in the air, we couldn't get warm, doors - that were stiff and difficult to open - were swinging open. The prover looking after the fire pulled the wood out of the burner to check whether the wood was wet (it wasn't), and - even though it had been burning a little, the wood was cold. We felt uncomfortable and afraid. It was a palpable feeling. It was particularly noticed given that we had had a really lovely day together.

It was also noted by some provers that this is a remedy for those that are working to darker agendas whilst presenting themselves as wayshowers or bringers of light - the darkness in disguise. This is a remedy that can help us to identify those people more easily.

Struggle between Light and Darkness

Corporate Greed

We talked about manipulative sales and the push to do or say anything to drive sales - not that sales or marketing themselves are an issue; just that they are a tool that can be used with the energy and intention of the user - some use sales authentically and with love, others as a manipulation for their own ends, praying on people's difficulties with making decisions.

We talked about how Dr Richard Horton, Editor-in-Chief of the Lancet for over 25 years famous quote: "The case against science is straightforward: much of the scientific literature, perhaps half, may simply be untrue. Afflicted by studies with small sample sizes, tiny effects, invalid exploratory analyses, and flagrant conflicts of interest, together with an obsession for pursuing fashionable trends of dubious importance, science has taken a turn towards darkness."

The example of Vioxx was shared. Vioxx (generic name: rofecoxib) was a popular prescription nonsteroidal anti-inflammatory drug (NSAID) in the US, manufactured by Merck & Co. Estimates suggest that between 88,000 and 140,000 cases of serious heart disease were caused by Vioxx in the US during its time on the market (1999–2004), and that the serious risks of heart disease and strokes caused by it were known by Merck as early as 2000.

We also talked about how the new weight loss drug ozempic (semaglutide) carries a boxed warning due the risk of cancer found in animal studies.

Lack of Empathy

Building on the previous key themes, this remedy may be useful for those with a lack of empathy for their actions towards others.

Disconnection to Connection

We discussed the roll out of AI, and tech generally, as having the risks associated with them of disconnection. They are a tool and can be applied with connection in mind, however they also can bring great disconnection. We are so used to having answers at the instant press of a button, that we aren't so easily learning information that we can *retain,* which was discussed in the group.

Some provers discussed how a lot of people give their power away to others, or to AI (which can make mistakes) and so we can lose our connection to our discernment - which helps make us powerful (and sovereign).

This is also very much a remedy for those feeling disconnection. The Torus remedy invites a weaving of the different aspects that make up the totality of a person - in Goethe's terms, the *Körper* (body), *Gemut,* (mind), *Seele* (soul) and *Geist* (spirit) as described in the introductory writings of this book. Where there is a gap between the mind (what the ego wants to do and says is OK) and what the spirit invites (that higher part of us that knows what the most loving action is) is where dissonance and disconnection form - when we act in a way that isn't in alignment with a higher part of us.

Healing

One prover experienced a healing with someone she had had a difficult ending with a year previously. She said: "[The person] has just got in touch just to say thinking about you......feels like a lovely "sealing it in" - bringing a completeness.". It felt healing.

Another prover described situations of abandonment, feeling lost. This is a remedy that can help people find their way forward again.

One prover talked about the "womb-like space" that emerged and was deeply healing.

Protection

Several provers noticed feeling "a lack of protection", which came in as the proving progressed.

This remedy brings in protection where it is needed.

Mental / Emotional Symptoms

Fear
Lack of protection
Sense of being manipulated
Frustration
Annoyance at every trifle
Annoyed by sounds; quietness needed
Division (from self or within a group)
Lack of cohesiveness
Tense feeling
Anger
Rage
Distracted
Difficulty making decisions
Feeling exposed
Corruption
Greed
Manipulation of truth - for those manipulating, as well as those being manipulated
Difficulties identifying own resonance and truth
Giving power away easily to others
Feeling disconnected
Feeling far away from others

Disillusionment with systems
Lack of empathy
Lack of trust
Inner division: "I am good / I am bad"
Self-judgment
Lack of self-love
Body dysmorphia
Feeling hollow and empty
Grief
Exclusion
Abandonment
Feeling lost
Addictions
Fear of falling asleep
Fear of the dark or being alone at night
Feeling as though someone is watching during sleep
Eating disorders
Anorexia
Bulimia
Compulsive eating
Cutting
Restlessness - tired but cannot rest

Physical Particular Symptoms

Head

Headache - pounding across forehead
Migraine - feeling as though head being attacked

Eyes

Sore eyes
Redness

Ears

Sensitivity to sounds
Annoyed by sounds; desire for reverence, quietness needed

Nose

Extreme sensitivity to all smells
Smell of tobacco causes either extreme dislike, or desire for cigarettes

Mouth & Teeth

Cavities
Tooth decay

Throat

Lump in throat
Clearing throat repeatedly, but doesn't clear what needs clearing
Sore throat, red
Inflammation

Lungs & Breathing

Shallow breathing
Difficulties with breathing - can't get enough air in
Feeling of weight on chest, affecting breathing
Pressure on chest
Sharp pain on inhalation

Heart

Athersclerosis
Blocked arteries

Heavy feeling in heart
Sinking feeling in heart
Palpitations
Inflammation

Digestion

Microbiome in disarray
Dysbiosis
Gastritis
Inflammation
Ulcerative Colitis
Ulcers

Stomach

Helicobacter pylori
Ulcers

Liver

Toxic overload
Sluggish liver
Fatty liver disease
Cholangitis
Cirrhosis

Kidneys

Inflammation
Nephritis
Glomerulonephritis

Bladder

Cystitis

Female Reproductive

Protects mother during pregnancy
Endometriosis
Sex addiction

Male Reproduction

Sex addiction

Back & Limbs

Bad pain in left shoulder - may extend to tension in head

Skin

Fungal infections - eg fungal toe nails

Sleep

Disturbed sleep
Unsettled sleep

Dreams

Dreams of being abandoned, no resources, lost
Dreams of hooded, dark or unsettling figures
Fearful dreams - of being chased, or being attacked, or attacking someone else
Dreams of death or dying
Dreams of addictions

Nightmares

Body Temperature

Extreme cold
Shivering
Cannot get warm

Food & Drink

Food addiction
Loss of appetite
Eating disorders

Energy Levels

Low energy, but has difficulties resting
Fragmented energy
Lack of motivation
Drained - as though being drained by a situation or person(s) or an energy

Spiritual

Dark magic being used
Entities / attachments
Shadow work, confronting own shadow, fears, darkness
Light vs dark battle, deception disguising light
Spiritual protection: closing doors, womb-like protection
Torus field, geometric shapes, energetic fields being warped
Energies that need Transmutation
Spiritual cleansing and protection practices
Addictions

Clinical

Inflammation - anywhere in the body
Smoking
Addictions
Dysbiosis
Nephritis
Glomerulonephritis
Liver, sluggish
Ulcers
Fatty liver disease
Cholangitis
Cirrhosis

Remedy Affinities

Amethyst
Anacardium
Ayahuasca
Bryonia
Carcinosin
Nitric Acid
Kali
Medorrhinum
Obsidian
Staphysagria
Stramonium
Syphilinum
Tabernanthe Iboga (Declan Hammond)
Vector Equilibrium
Vernix Caseosa

Prescribing Notes

1) Torus combines wonderfully with Vector Equilibrium - I tend to prescribe both together. The complement each other beautifully - Torus repairs the energy field, and Vector Equilibrium returns to balance and centre. I tend to give a 30c daily when needed.

Case Studies

1) JP - Fungal Toes

I have tried every single indicated therapeutic, constitutional and miasmatic remedy for a patient with a fungal infection on three toes on the left foot, including the big toe. Nothing has worked until I used a blend with Torus in it. JP has has tried every natural product on the market, used tea tree, lemon, vinegar, a blend with walnut and wormwood tincture in it, and other natural products over prolonged periods of time. Nothing has worked. It has affected the patient's toes for over 10 years.

I made the following combination, and whilst it has taken time, and needs to be taken 2-3 times a day, at the time of publication, following 2 months' use, healthy nail has been growing back from the root, and half of the big toe now is clear of fungus.

Torus / Vector Equilibrium / Bosnian Pyramid of the Sun / Antimonium tartaricum / Thuja 200c 2-3 times daily

(Bosnian Pyramid of the Sun has an anti-fungal aspect to its picture).

It may be that increasing potencies over time is needed too.

2) GL - ADHD, autism & burnout

GL a 45 year old Black British woman with ADHD and autism, a history of long term burnout, fibroids, hormonal dysregulation, and personal and generational trauma consistent with CPTSD.

She has used homeopathy as her primary mode of healing for approximately six years.

Her life involves sustained cognitive, emotional, and relational demand. Alongside work and study, she is highly creative, and loves to dance, sing and write. She maintains close relationships and regularly holds emotional and mental space for others in both her personal life and professional roles as a qualified mental health practitioner and holistic energy worker.

This level of engagement creates continuous demand switching, layered cognitive load, and difficulty fully powering down. For a neurodivergent nervous system shaped by trauma, fatigue is not a lack of motivation but the cost of sustained integration and meaning-making.

Rather than aiming to resolve or eliminate symptoms, sacred geometry homeopathic remedies Vector Equilibrium and Torus were used as supports for regulation and coherence within an already overloaded system.

Vector Equilibrium, understood in sacred geometry as equalised forces and zero-point balance, was experienced as a settling of internal competition. It did not sedate or energise, but supported a felt neutrality in which fewer internal demands competed for priority. Early observations included reduced urgency, quieter internal dialogue, and increased tolerance for ambiguity and unfinished tasks.

As this baseline stabilised, the Torus pattern, representing continuous circulation, inward gathering, and outward expression, was associated with improved flow. Energy levels did not increase, but energy distribution became more even. Creative work felt less all-or-nothing, emotional labour less depleting, and recovery following exertion more reliable. Burnout symptoms persisted but were less abrupt in their onset, with rest experienced as more restorative.

Overall, the experience was not of cure, but of reduced internal friction. Fatigue remained present, yet felt more organised and manageable.

This case suggests that the remedies Vector Equilibrium and Torus actively assist complex nervous systems in relating to their limits with greater flexibility and ease.

Vector Equilibrium

17 August 2025
Uluru National Park
Northern Territory
Australia

22 & 23 November 2025
USA & Canada (various locations)

29 & 30 November 2025
UK & Australia (various locations)

8 provers were involved with the first trituration, which took place in Australia. All 8 were women. This was triturated using the intuitive trituration method to a 13c, in view of Uluru. The trituration followed a once-in-a-lifetime experience of walking the 6km walk around Uluru.

There were further triturations to a 3c at the Golden Spiral International School of Homeopathy on two weekends in November 2025. Over 30 provers were present at each weekend. All participants on both weekends were women.

Vector Equilibrium

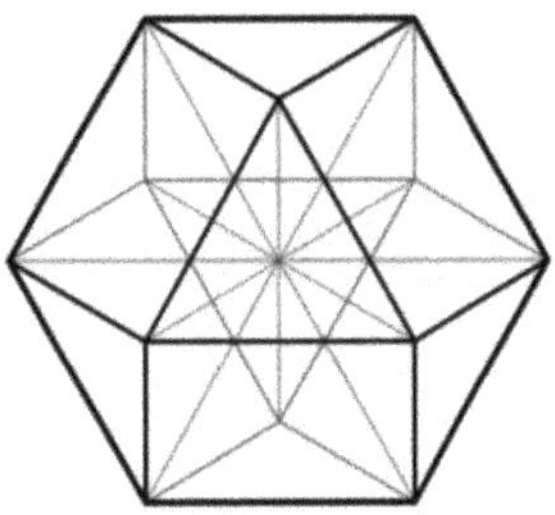

Vector Equilibrium emanates energy in twelve directions. R. Buckminster Fuller Vector Equilibrium described this as the first "Buckyball" - a "cosmic zero", in which, at its centre, is a primal emptiness & the normal laws of the space time continuum break down. It is a zone in which, according to Fuller, waves can pass through without interference. It holds the tension of the opposites and brings them together, so is a powerful symbol for moving from polarity or duality to unity at the centre.

There is a move from the opposing forces of push/pull, tension/compression to a central point of stillness.

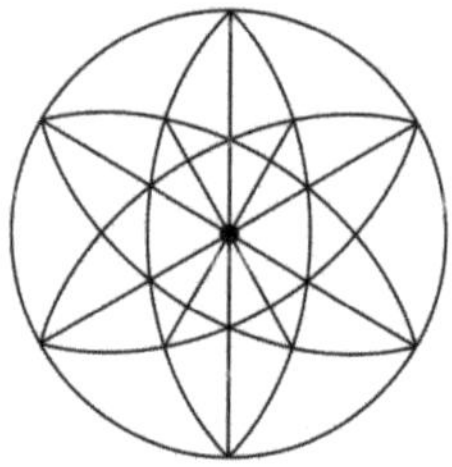

There are two states of the Vector Equilibrium: one comprised of lines (first image) which shows the structure of the vector equilibrium -or how the equilibrium is organised. The other state is a sphere (second image is a 2D visual of what becomes the third image - the sphere) - this is how the vector equilibrium flows, or is experienced.

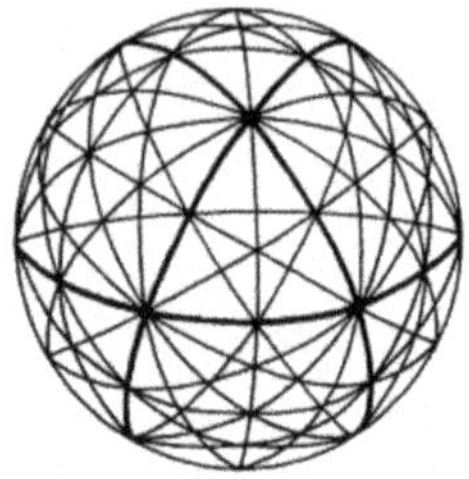

Fuller talked about how they were different states of the same thing. There is a something called the "jitterbug effect" which can be viewed visually online, where the vector equilibrium moves, expands and collapses, and as it does so, it transforms into the Platonic solid shapes: tetrahedron, octahedron and, icosahedron.

Another way of looking at vector equilibrium is that the image with the lines is the equilibrium we can measure, whereas the sphere is the equilibrium we can feel. Both have the same centre and the same balance; the movement from polarity to unity, duality to centre.

Ultimately, vector equilibrium equalises different (opposing) forces and brings us to zero-point balance,

Vector Equilibrium Homeopathic Remedy™

Key Themes

Wholeness
Belonging - to self
Inclusion / Exclusion
Nature's Interconnectedness
Duality to Unity
Resonance of Calm & Balance
Community, Connection & Support
Expressing truths, needs & desires
Healing
Honouring Ancient Wisdoms and Traditions
Letting Go
Hope
Happiness
Mitochondria

Wholeness

A central theme of the remedy is the movement toward *wholeness of self*. There was a sense of completeness - and the peace that this brings. There was a total acceptance of the self, and then in relation to each other. It brought such peace to everyone.

The provers were able to move from any self-doubt and inadequacy toward self-acceptance, confidence, and embodiment. One prover shared: "I was born to do this. I can do this. I am good enough." Another shared: "Trust in yourself. You don't need validation or approval to you you can do it, be it, are it."

The wholeness, particularly in Australia was experienced as a whole group also - a cohesiveness, and wholeness together; a oneness.

With the wholeness was a sense of safety, self-reliance, and the balance between responsibility and freedom. There was an understanding that it was "ok to have fun and make mistakes" - that there was a safe and wide space for each individual to explore, to try things out, free of fear of judgement about whether something would work out or not. It felt safe to just "be", to explore, to try new things.

The energy was very much how children can play without intervention, just been witnessed with love, within a playroom, whilst they are exploring, having fun, being held safely as they do so.

Belonging

In the wholeness is a sense of belonging to oneself - there was no longer a need to seek belonging externally because it was felt internally. And yet the provers, particularly in the Australian trituration felt such a strong sense of belonging to each other. Yet it felt like it came from a place of belonging to ourselves first - an ease and comfort with ourselves.

As one prover said: "I can belong anywhere if I am whole, if I belong to me, if I accept myself."

Inclusion / Exclusion

Several provers experienced a feeling of exclusion or inclusion. As one prover shared: "Feel outside, disconnected, cut off, left out, outside looking in. Want to feel included, good enough, wanted but don't. Feelings of immense sadness and longing for something, to be part of something, feeling I"m not wanted. Exclusion to inclusion......separation is an illusion created by fear. Releasing of the hold of the ego over the mind - the ego's hold over the mind is slipping away. Labyrinth movie, Sara to the Goblin King: 'You have no power over me'.....Not leaving anyone out."

One talked about feeling the "communal circle" and the feeling of "being held".

Nature's Interconnectedness

There was a true appreciation of the natural world around us. At one point a prover was focused on a standing tap that was dripping water, and made attempt to switch the tap off (to conserve water).

Two of us had stopped to watch ants interacting during the walk around Uluru before the trituration, it was such an adorable experience. There was a pumpkin seed on the ground that one ant was trying desperately hard to move, and it looked like it was trying to persuade the other ants to come and help, but they were focused on a chocolate chip on the ground. The one ant wouldn't give up, he kept trying and trying all on his own to move the pumpkin seed as though he had found the greatest prize.

We talked about fungi and the mycelial networks, how trees communicate with each other, and desert oak trees in Australia - they are an iconic, slow-growing tree found in central deserts, known for their deep roots (30x its height) and their ability to reach water. Some trees live for over 1000 years.

This is a remedy that speaks to the interconnectedness of the entire ecosystem that we are - including in our bodies, with our microbiome - and the ecosystem's ability to heal itself.

As one prover said: "The nature around Chernobyl has healed itself thanks to the black fungus, cryptococcus neoformans, which has literally been mopping up the radiation! David Attenborough was filmed there, and when you see it, there is so much vegetation - trees and plants growing through and around the deserted buildings, with deer and other wildlife wandering through it. Nature has found a way to bring the area back to healing and balance!"

One of the teachings I share with students at the Golden Spiral International School of Homeopathy® is that we are a living expression of an ecosystem: we aren't just one entity; a person. We are an ecosystem and expression of that ecosystem. We think that our vital force is the expression of a singularity; the person that we are. I really believe that our vital force is a the expression of the ecosystem - a collective voice expressing the interconnected ecosystem we are made of - humans, bacteria, fungi, protozoa, viruses, parasites. Our vital force is not the expression of a soloist, but rather the collective expression of a beautiful orchestra; a symphony. If any one part of the orchestra is off-key, the vital force of the orchestra is affected.

Vector Equilibrium speaks to the balance between all members of our microbiome; our ecosystem. If there is an imbalance, it seeks to bring us back to balance where there is a place and space for every part of the ecosystem in balance with every other part of it.

We also talked about a video that had gone viral shortly before the Uluru adventure - of a woman standing next to a tree, with a branch close to her face, and her repeatedly saying "touch my face" to the tree, and the branch moving to touch her face. Some of the provers tried it under a tree in front of Uluru and it worked! We were really celebrating being part of a larger connected Oneness with nature.

Several provers described hearing the sound vibrations of nature around us, including hearing the water vibrations through the trees, the songs sung by the winds, the sun, and the sounds of wildlife and the natural world around us.

Duality to Unity

Vector equilibrium helps us to move from duality to unity. This is represented in many aspects: left and right, yin and yang, masculine and feminine balance, control and surrender, collapse and creation, inclusion and exclusion.

Balance is also expressed in natural cycles: we talked about fire stick farming for ecosystem balance, breathing in and out, holding and releasing. During the trituration, a prover noticed the "resistance to mix, two parts equally important", another noted that the "left and right integrated... masculine and feminine." A third stated that "it came together instantly when I lifted the pestle and stopped forcing it."

Restoration of Calm & Balance

During the triturations in Australia (at Uluru), and in the USA and Canada, there was a clear calm within the group throughout the trituration. This is what Vector Equilibrium brings us to - peace , calm and stillness in the centre. We were completely in balance with one another, each being equally as valued as the other, and each having her place and space.

In the UK & Australia trituration during November 2025, there were experiences of the time before we come to calm. There were repeated experiences of chaos - family, time pressure, confusion, disorder, noise, emotional overwhelm - preceding sudden calm, clarity, renewal and flow. One prover said "The morning was very chaotic... then suddenly everyone went to their activity." Another said: "Complete chaos, I'm late... yet I feel this calmness inside." One more also described a "chaos before the calm." Another shared: "Chaos, destruction - building up then breaking down.", and saw an amphitheatre collapsing. Another described the "order among chaos"; the "beautiful disorder".

One prover in the in-person trituration shared "the beautiful sounds of the group almost harmonising at points and complete chaos at other points which felt distracting."

Where there is a lack of balance, the Vector Equilibrium restores this. We have already explored this in relation to the microbiome and biological ecosystems. This is also applicable to other aspects of life, and the systems we find ourselves in; from family systems, to organisational systems.

Community, Connection & Support

I have described how we were completely in balance with one another, each being equally as valued as the other, and each having her place and space in the trituration at Uluru.

There was a real sense of deep connection with one another; truly supporting each other - not from a place of trying to fix or solve problems or co-dependence - more a gentle coming alongside one another, trusting completely that the person knew what they needed at any one time, and being happy and willing to support as and when needed, but in a light touch way. It felt so balanced, and respectful.

This remedy also made it easier to receive support. As one prover stated: "I allowed support even if it was not perfect." Another noticed "Support appears the moment it is allowed."

There was a lot of love felt for one another. As one prover said: "Love. Heart expansion, allowing love in, learning to trust with the heart, love is the key to all."

Expressing truths, needs & desires

Speaking up in order to express needs and receive support is also important in this remedy. As one prover shared: "I called my dad and had a chat with him regarding an issue and it got a little messy being of a certain generation. However my father apologised to me twice and I actually felt heard. I then had an emotional clearing and felt a freedom and control of myself which I have never felt before. [Usually when} speaking [up] I will wheeze and have trouble breathing. However when speaking to my sister and dad I was clear as anything no wheeze or struggle breathing just saying what I needed too. That's the first thing I realised and I was in shock as this is not normal for me."

Healing

We discussed vibrational medicine, healing frequencies, and subtle healing practices that are tied to nature's rhythms.

This remedy welcomes a reconnection with these.

Honouring Ancient Wisdoms & Traditions

As I shared in the Vesica Piscis proving, this is another remedy that connects us with the teachings of Francesca Mason Boring, who teaches how Indigenous cultures place meaning and connection at the centre of life. Keeping a connection to higher wisdom and knowledge ensures there is always a balance with nature in life. The Western world places materialism at the centre of life, and this creates distortion and a lack of balance - this takes away from connection at the centre, and to duality and polarity. Like Vesica

Piscis, Vector Equilibrium restores a relationship with connection and meaning at the centre of life.

During the proving, we discussed the passing on of knowledge that Indigenous cultures practice - how cultural wisdom is shared during walks and in connection with nature. We talked about the honouring of "men's business" and "women's business". When walking around Uluru, there are areas where it's possible to come right up close and touch her, and we are allowed to take photos. There are areas where we are not allowed to take photos, where we are directed far from the rock - this is because those areas are for sacred ceremonies including some areas for men's business and some areas for women's business. These might seem dualistic in their nature, but they are simply an honouring that, once they happen, allow a welcome back to centre together from a place of balance.

We talked about fire stick farming, promised marriages and also skin names.

Indigenous Australians are born with a skin name based on their parents. It is usually seen as their middle name. "It gives them an immediate relationship within their community and their country, relating to he landscape, wildlife and their associated Dreamings.....Depending on an [Indigenous] person's skin name they have immediate and predefined relationships with each of the other skin names. These relationships are complex and will dictate much of daily life including the important relationship of who they can marry.[46]

The importance of respecting and maintaining cultural heritage and natural wisdom came through strongly in this proving, as

46 https://artark.com.au/pages/aboriginal-skin-names-1#:~:text=Aboriginal people are born with,of who they can marry.

Indigenous cultures have at their centre balance.

Letting Go

This remedy helps us to let go of what no longer serves us - whether it is objects, patterns, roles, relationships, beliefs.

One prover lost her sunglasses. On reflection she realised she was shedding what no longer serves. Another said "We are custodians [of objects] rather than owners."

The letting go can be uncomfortable at times - Vector Equilibrium us always seeking balance. Sometimes it's difficult to let go of what we have in our lives, because it is what we are used to, however in seeking to establish calm, connection and unity, the letting go can be necessary.

Several provers were experiencing constipation during the proving, which for each was not a normal experience for them - a further example of the need for letting go.

Hope

We discussed pollution, 5G, radiation, and fungi's role in healing the planet. There was a recognition of human impact and the need for sustainable practices (for example fire farming as part of maintaining ecological balance).

We discussed some of the projects being developed by young people that are clearing our world of pollution, or helping others, such as the discovery fungi that eat plastics in the oceans. We felt optimistic about young generations and scientific advances nurturing the planet's future.

These are further examples of how we are moving from chaos, lack

of connection, disunity, duality - back to centre, calm, stillness and equilibrium.
Where the remedy Ayahuasca brings us a light to light our way forward out of the darkness, Vector Equilibrium welcomes a gentle hope for the future.

Happiness

There was a collective experience of happiness when we made this remedy by Uluru. There was a lot of laughter, lightness, giggling during the trituration. Even in the more serious conversations, there wasn't a heaviness, just a matter-of-fact sharing. Life felt easy and happy.

Mitochondria

Vector Equlibrium has an affinity with mitochondria. Like conception occurs because all of the forces of the Universe come to a single point in time a space; a convergence - a singularity - the mitochondria are the key to successful conception. Mitochondria do not just produce energy through the breakdown of adenosine triphosphate (ATP) into adenosine diphosphate (ADP), releasing a phosphate. Mitochondria also produce *water* as biochemist Carrie Bennett teaches. Water, as we are discovering thanks to the work of Veda Austin and others, is literally Source within the body.

Vector Equilibrium brings all elements to one point for the expression of creation. Mitochondria - originally of bacterial origin - make this possible in our bodies.

Mental / Emotional Symptoms

Polarity
Disunity
Disagreements
Imbalances
Chaos
Lack of peace
Out of balance masculine or feminine
Stress
Loneliness
Lack of support
Depression
Unhappiness
Conflicting pressures
Torn between situations or demands
Dogma
Difficulties making decisions
Lack of safety
Lack of accountability
Fear of making mistakes
Feeling wrong
Inner conflict
Uncertain of identity
Spark of first love, flutter of excitement
Difficulties letting go of what is no longer needed or what no longer serves
Too much materialism
Custodianship rather than ownership
Feeling stuck in the middle
Weary
Desire for calm

Feeling tired after work or ritual
Dysregulated nervous system
A need to feel supported and soothed
Bullying - for those experiencing bullying or perpetuating it
Desire to feel happy and connected
Disconnected from nature
Concern about radiation, pollution, and impact on health
Health anxiety
Anxieties about the destruction of the planet
Need for laughter; not much lightness or laughter in the person's life
Shyness in groups - difficulties speaking up and sharing
Imbalances in relationships
Jealousy
Women and men uncertain about their roles in their relationships
Feelings of inadequacy
Comparing self against others
Lack of trust in oneself
Cutting

Physical Particular Symptoms

Head

Headache
Headache over right eyebrow
Head feels large, expanded
Overthinking
Brain does not switch off
Encephalitis
Heaviness of head

Eyes

Difficulties focusing
Astigmatism

Blurred vision
Eyes stinging
Sharp stabbing pain - right eye
Feeling pressure on third eye (in between my eyes)

Ears

Sensitive hearing
Tinnitus
Blocked ear - right

Nose

Sensitive to smell of pollution

Mouth & Teeth

Out of balance oral microbiome
Overuse of antibacterial mouthwashes and toothpastes

Throat

Difficulties speaking up
Shyness
Lump in the throat when trying to speak
Laryngitis
Inflammation
Difficulties swallowing, better warm drinks
Hot, dry throat

Lungs & Breathing

Shallow breathing
Irregular breathing
Asthma

Tight chest, feeling anxious
Struggling to breathe
Heaviness on the chest
Gasping for air.
Tar in the lungs

Heart

Irregular heartbeat
Angina

Digestion

Constipation
Dysbiosis (gut microbiome out of balance)
Crohn's disease
Sour smelling stools
Greenish stools

Stomach

Heliobacter pylori
Inflammation
Acidity
Reflux
Eructations - with sour or acid taste

Liver

Sluggish liver

Bladder

Frequency of urination
Urgency of urination

Cystitis

Female Reproductive

Pregnant women - start taking one month before birth, calls in support for the birth
Support during fertility treatment
Weak or irregular ovulation
Low progesterone
Too much or too little testosterone
Hormone imbalances

Male Reproduction

Low sperm motility
Too much or too little testosterone

Back & Limbs

Inflamed spot on muscle, worse pressure, better stretching
Cramp
Back aching over right ribs
Feeling of cold down the spine
Shoulder tension

Skin

Dermatitis
Allergic reactions
Red, sore or dry patches, difficult to heal
Sore skin, worse washing in warm water, better in cold water
Difficulty retaining moisture in skin

Physical General Symptoms

Sleep

Feeling tired often, possibly after ritual or work
Difficulties falling asleep due to overthinking
Waking early, difficulty falling asleep due to overthinking

Body Temperature

Extremes of body temperature - too hot or too cold

Food & Drink

Very thirsty

Energy Level

Need to "power on"
Stamina - has stamina or needs stamina
Feeling tired after certain tasks

Clinical

Crohn's Disease
Autoimmune conditions
Helicobacter pylori
Adrenal fatigue
Hormone imbalances

Spiritual

Seed of Life symbolism, ancient bacterial and human connection
Perfection of self, natural orchestration of life
Uluru's heartbeat, spiritual vibrations through nature
Magpie as messenger of positive and negative aspects
Passing on of wisdom through natural sounds and group rituals
Indigenous cultural knowledge, skin name promises, family roles
Kabbalah references, big bang, cosmic unity
Spiritual balance in community, equality, and connection
Purity of life
Love

Remedy Affinities

Arsenicum album
Birdsong
Dodona
Golden Spiral
Lycopodium
Lotus
Nat mur
Thymus gland
Vesica Piscis

Prescribing Notes

1) This remedy works through the entire family system - when one person takes it, other members of the family may also feel it.

Case Studies

1) GL - ADHD, autism & burnout

GL a 45 year old Black British woman with ADHD and autism, a history of long term burnout, fibroids, hormonal dysregulation, and personal and generational trauma consistent with CPTSD.

She has used homeopathy as her primary mode of healing for approximately six years.

Her life involves sustained cognitive, emotional, and relational demand. Alongside work and study, she is highly creative, and loves to dance, sing and write. She maintains close relationships and regularly holds emotional and mental space for others in both her personal life and professional roles as a qualified mental health practitioner and holistic energy worker.

This level of engagement creates continuous demand switching, layered cognitive load, and difficulty fully powering down. For a neurodivergent nervous system shaped by trauma, fatigue is not a lack of motivation but the cost of sustained integration and meaning-making.

Rather than aiming to resolve or eliminate symptoms, sacred geometry homeopathic remedies Vector Equilibrium and Torus were used as supports for regulation and coherence within an already overloaded system.

Vector Equilibrium, understood in sacred geometry as equalised forces and zero-point balance, was experienced as a settling of internal competition. It did not sedate or energise, but supported a felt neutrality in which fewer internal demands competed for priority. Early observations included reduced urgency, quieter internal dialogue, and increased tolerance for ambiguity and unfinished tasks.

As this baseline stabilised, the Torus pattern, representing continuous circulation, inward gathering, and outward expression, was associated with improved flow. Energy levels did not increase, but energy distribution became more even. Creative work felt less all-or-nothing, emotional labour less depleting, and recovery following exertion more reliable. Burnout symptoms persisted but were less abrupt in their onset, with rest experienced as more restorative.

Overall, the experience was not of cure, but of reduced internal friction. Fatigue remained present, yet felt more organised and manageable.

This case suggests that the remedies Vector Equilibrium and Torus actively assist complex nervous systems in relating to their limits with greater flexibility and ease.

Part 3

Platonic Solids Remedies

The Platonic Solids

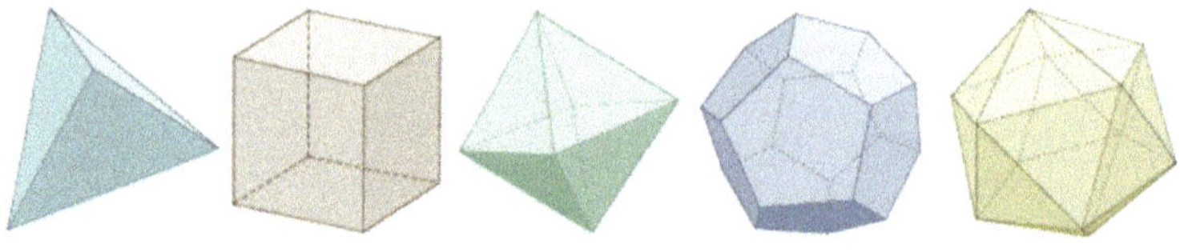

The Platonic solids were originally five unique, perfectly symmetrical 3D shapes (tetrahedron, cube, octahedron, dodecahedron, icosahedron). They represent all of the ways in which the Universe itself exists and is structured.

They are named after Plato (c. 428–348 BCE), the Ancient Greek philosopher who had been taught by Socrates, and was a teacher of Aristotle.

Their key feature is that each one is made of a polygon shape (in other words, a 2D shape with equal length sides eg an equilateral triangle or a square) that has become a 3D shape. So 4 sides of an equilateral triangle forms a pyramid (tetrahedron), 6 sides of a square forms a cube, and so on.

These are the only 5 shapes that are possible with polygons. These are names after Plato, the Ancient Greek teacher who linked them with the 5 classical elements, fire, earth, air, water and spirit (or Universe).

They are said to actually have been discovered by Pythagoras (c. 570–490 BCE),, however Pythagoras hadn't done very much with them, and when Plato discovered them, and then linked them with the elements, they emerged into the collective consciousness.

The Platonic solids demonstrate the *structure* to the Universe, and the Sacred Geometry (eg Golden Spiral, Flower of Life, Vector Equilibrium), is how *energy flows* within it.

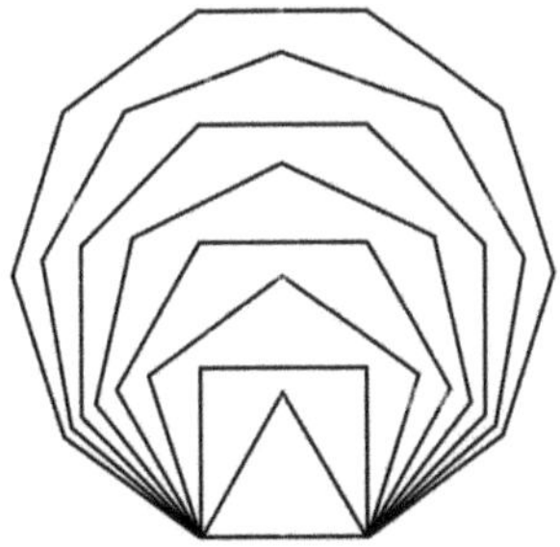

I see them as the Platonic solids being like the masculine, holding structure, seeing the beauty of the feminine creative energy (the Sacred Geometry) that flows within.

Metatron's Cube is known by some as the 6th Platonic solid - however it isn't actually a polygon itself. It contains all of the 5 original Platonic solids.

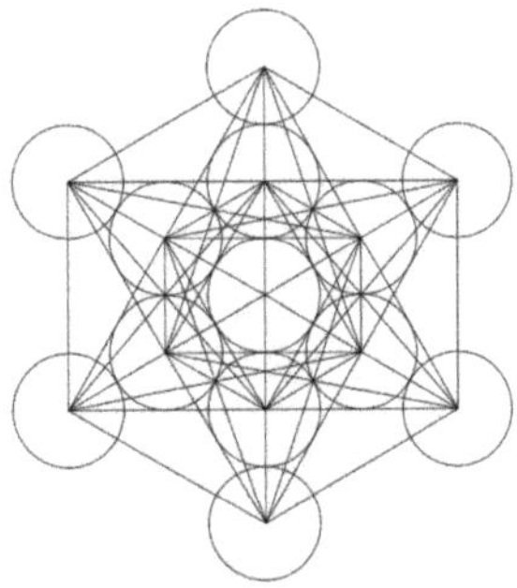

Archangel Metatron is the Archangel who is said to be able to explain divine science, the divine electron, all of the levels of existence and form - as has been written about in the 1973 channelled book by J.J. Hurtak the *Keys of Enoch*.

Metatron's Cube is said to contain all of the geometry relating the the structure of the Universe, and of all reality.

Tetrahedron

16 December 2025
East Sussex
England

This remedy was triturated from an essence prepared by the author using the intuitive trituration method. The substance was triturated to 13c in October 2025, with a follow-up proving conducted on 16 December 2025.

Triturated and proved by the author.

Tetrahedron

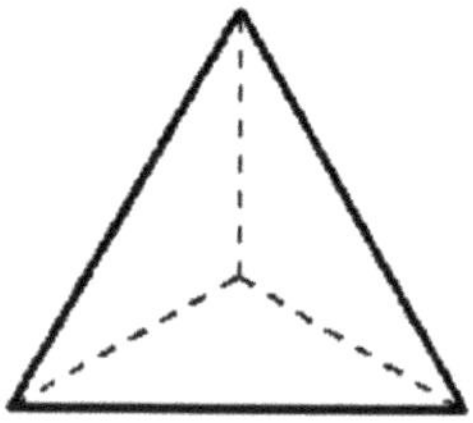

The Tetrahedron is a four-sided pyramid. It is the simplest of the Platonic solids. It represents the element of Fire.

The tetrahedron also represents willpower, action, motivation, knowledge, and the sacred masculine. The tetrahedron (pyramid pointing up) is a masculine energy - and looks symbolically like an activated expression of the male reproductive system. It combines with the pyramid pointing down (representing the feminine, like the upside down triangle shape of the women's reproductive system), to form the star tetrahedron.

Metaphysically, the tetrahedron can connect us with the qualities of the masculine, including decision-making, logical thinking and being in the energy of doing.

Tetrahedron Homeopathic Remedy™

Key Themes

Taking Action
Motivation
New Ideas, Solutions & Progress
Completion
Communication
Virility
Power, Confidence & Assertiveness
Competition
I AM presence

Taking Action

This is a remedy that called us into action. During the proving, I needed to move, one walking around the room constantly whilst talking - it wasn't at a fast pace, both the walking and talking were at a "normal" pace. I felt so much energy running through me, that I didn't feel able to sit down. It was a comfortable experience of walking, not frenzied in any way. I was reminded of my son when he was small. I used to be in awe at all of his energy. He didn't have ADHD, but he just couldn't stop moving and just doing things when he was awake. He always wanted to be running, climbing trees, out exploring the world. I just couldn't understand it. During the proving I felt like that - like I saw in him when he was small I just wanted to be out there doing things. I had all this energy and I want to get things done.

Motivation

Along with the energy of taking action, there is an increase in motivation - a desire to do things; to get going. I had a desire to go through paperwork, and clear it, which is unusual for me.

I also felt a desire to wash the windows, which is not like me either.

New Ideas, Solutions & Progress

Inherent in taking action and having more motivation, is being able to make progress. As well as making progress in areas that have stalled, there is also an element of making progress with problems, or ideas that have paused or become stuck. New solutions may present themselves.

I experienced many new ideas coming to me, and felt more positive, hopeful and optimistic about a situation I needed to find a way forward with. I felt it would be easier to resolve than I had worried (which turned out to be the case).

Completion

This remedy has the energy within it to ensure tasks are seen through to completion. This may be a useful remedy for people who give up easily, or who start projects but rarely finish them.

I felt like I could accomplish tasks and see them through to completion even more quickly and easily than I would normally. .

Communication

I felt that it was easier to communicate than normal. I experienced greater loquacity, and less of a filter – an inner voice suggesting when to speak and when not to speak. I felt more confident expressing myself than usual. Like a whisper, almost not there at all. “No!” I want to say. “My voice matters! What I have to say counts! I matter! I have a voice! It's important I use it!”.”

This may be useful as a remedy for those who are shy, or who find it difficult speaking to other others.

In writing this, I am reminded of one theory of how pyramids have been used for communication with the stars. They amplify energy and beam it into the cosmos, according to some researchers. This remedy amplifiers our power, our energy, and our voice. I wonder if it would be useful in supporting not only communication with our fellow humans, but may also connect us with communication with the stars.

Virility

The masculine energy of taking action inherent in this remedy, and the element of fire and passion connects us also with the experience of virility. There may be an increased desire for sex, an increased appetite for sex and this is a useful remedy to consider for times of low sex drive, and impotence..

Power, Confidence & Assertiveness

I was reminded of a really important constellation that I was a part of. In it, I was invited to represent the consciousness of men. As soon as I stepped into the representation, I felt amazing. I felt unlike I had ever felt before as a woman, I felt like there was room for me - space for me to exist in the world. I felt like I could take up plenty of space, and that it was my right to do so. I felt unimpeded, as though there were no obstacles to my being able to take up any space.

There is a scene in the film *Barbie*, when Barbie starts to notice some uncomfortable feelings, she's never had these before and she voices this disquiet that is happening within her. She says: "I'm getting all these weird feelings - like fear, but there's no particular object?" A woman behind her overhears and tells her, "That's anxiety! I get that too."

"When I was representing men, I just had no anxiety. The anxiety of existence, was completely absent. I didn't even realise that I lived with it as a norm, a feeling that there wasn't a place for me in this world. But when representing the consciousness of men, it just wasn't there. It just was a truth that I exist and that there is a place for me in the world.

I felt powerful in ways I have never felt power before. I quickly realised that I could have anything that I wanted. And I also got to see the shadow side of this, which was that if anyone said no to me, I could if I wished just help myself anyway - because I could; because I was powerful. That was quite a sobering moment.

This remedy makes me feel powerful, like I felt then. This is a remedy for people who feel powerless.

I observed a powerfulness in how I was expressing myself; I felt I could do anything.

With the power is courage, from the perspective of the true meaning of courage - "with [the] whole heart".

There is a greater assertiveness in this remedy.

Competition

This is a remedy that helps people find the drive they need to move forward. However, it also will bring balance where competitiveness has gone out of balance. The pyramid is made of polygons, which means equal lengths of sides, and equal angles between the sides.

Equality and balance are inherent in polygons and in these remedies. I was reminded of how a little competition can be healthy, it can help to push people forwards, and to motivate them. It's when it goes out of balance that it's a problem. This is a remedy to return to balance what may have gone out of balance.

I AM presence

Our "I AM presence" refers to our Divinity. It reminds us of the God/Divine/Source aspect that resides within each of us. The "I AM" refers to the truth that we exist. It is a very empowering statement. This remedy connect us with the energy of our "I AM presence" – the confidence in ourselves that we matter, that we are here, that we have a place and space in this world, and a purpose too.

Mental / Emotional Symptoms

Feelings of inadequacy
Comparing self against others
Lack of trust in oneself
No or low confidence
No or low motivation
Distracted easily
Difficulties completing tasks or goals
Feeling powerless
Wanting to hide away
Shyness
Feeling stuck
Too many problems
Can't find a way out of problems
Searching for answers, solutions
Difficulties making decisions
No or low sexual desire

Lack of self-belief
Feeling that they don't matter
No or low drive
Lack of self-belief
Muddled
Poor memory
Can't think straight
Have given up
Poor boundaries
Lack of assertiveness

Physical Particular Symptoms

Head

Foggy head
Muddled easily
Confusion
Hard to think
Difficulties making decisions

Eyes

Difficulties focusing
Astigmatism
Blurred vision

Ears

Itchy ear - left

Throat

Difficulties speaking up
Shyness

Lump in the throat when trying to speak

Lungs & Breathing

Out of breath easily

Heart

Weak pulse
Weak heart

Digestion

Constipation
Incomplete evacuation

Liver

Sluggish liver

Bladder

Tenesmus
Urinary retention
Bladder not emptying fully
Cystitis
Burning on urination

Female Reproductive

Low sex drive

Male Reproduction

Low sex drive

Impotence

Back & Limbs

Stiffness in joints
Slowness in movements
Rheumatoid Arthritis
Stiffness, better movement

Skin

Eczema - burning sensation on skin
Sensation as though skin is on fire
Acne
Pimples with burning sensation

Physical General Symptoms

Sleep

Oversleeping
Too much sleep - leaves person feeling sluggish

Body Temperature

Extremes of body temperature - too hot or too cold

Food & Drink

Thirsty
Desire for lemonade

Energy Level

Low energy

Clinical

Rheumatoid Arthritis
Inflammation
Pain

Spiritual

"I AM" presence
Lack of purpose & direction in life
Soul's journey
Feels that they do not matter
Transmutation
Boundaries
Not being held back anymore
Freedom to express oneself - to open one's heart
Courage ("with whole heart")

Remedy Affinities

Ambra grisea
Birdsong
Dodona
Golden Spiral
Orange
Lycopodium
Metatron's Cube
Milky Way
Red
Rhus toe
Ruta
Sepia

Hexahedron

17 December 2025
East Sussex
England

This remedy was triturated from an essence prepared by the author using the intuitive trituration method. The substance was triturated to 13c in October 2025, with a follow-up proving conducted on 17 December 2025.

Triturated and proved by the author.

Hexahedron

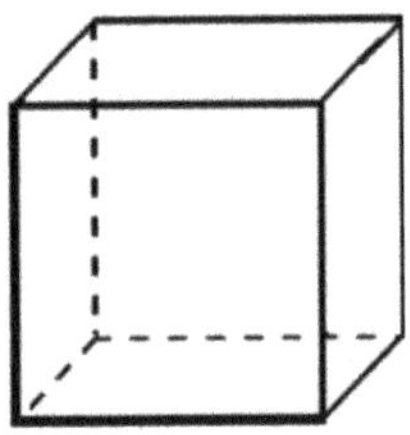

The Hexahedron is a six-sided cube. It represents the element of Earth.

The hexahedron represents stability, grounding, and structure. It also represents our connection to nature and the physical world - to our foundations and to mass. It is often linked to the Root Chakra.

Hexahedron Homeopathic Remedy™

Key Themes

Home and Belonging
Connection with Nature
Stability
Grounding
Safety & Protection

Manifestation & Materialisation
Structure
Community
Warmth & Contentment

Home and Belonging

Home is an important key theme for this remedy. We also see home as important in relation to the Pleiades homeopathic remedy too. With the Hexahedron, the focus is on the physical home; our physical home on Earth. With the Pleiades homeopathic remedy, there is a reference to our home in the stars. With the Hexahedron, it is our physical home - the one where we feel safe, secure, and stable.

I felt an even bigger urge to wash the windows than during the Tetrahedron proving, It came from a different space however. This time I wanted to wash the windows because I want to feel pride in my home. I love my home, I am grateful for it and I wanted to honour and look after my home. When I proved Tetrahedron, I wanted to wash the windows so that I could see clearly, as though this gave me a sense of direction and clear vision. With this remedy [Hexahedron], I was appreciating the beauty of my home, and wanting to keep it that way. I have never enjoyed cleaning windows, so this was a surprise.

I was reminded of the proving of Dodona when I developed a really odd desire to iron everything in sight - until that point in time, I hadn't loved ironing. I was even ironing bedsheets! This remedy has a similar feeling of joy and pride in one's home and furnishings, and feeling comfortable within it.

There is also a strong feeling of belonging in one's home. With belonging comes a feeling of being able to relax, to regulate the nervous system – the phrase "put your feet up ", really showed itself in this remedy. I reflected on how when I think of my home, I just feel like I can relax in it. Put my feet up. Rest. It feels nice. I know where everything is, how everything works – it's my place and space. I know every inch of it, and it knows every inch of me. Our energy fills it, we are it. I felt even more appreciative of it and thankful for it in a whole new way. I felt lucky to have it.

Connection with Nature

An ideal home usually has green spaces around it. Trees, gardens, flowers - access to nature. Many homes have been built in the Western world with little connection to nature. Many people live in apartments without easy access to green spaces. I could really feel the green of my garden during the proving.

It felt like it was an even more vibrant green than I have ever seen before. I felt happy as I looked at it. I reflected on how many newer buildings, especially apartment blocks, are being designed with green spaces up the outer walls or on roof terraces - there is an understanding that we need to live in a way that is integrated with the natural world, not separate from it.

Stability

The cube itself is a stable structure. Stability is inherent within it. This showed itself during the proving. I noticed feeling settled. I didn't need to move around. I felt a desire to sit with a tree and meditate underneath it. I like the solidity of trees, the stability, the strength. They are strong. Immovable. Stable. I felt strong and stable and from this relaxed.

When we feel relaxed, and stable, our nervous system regulates, if it has been dysregulated. This is a remedy that brings stability (and safety) that helps our nervous system regulate.

Grounding

This remedy is a deeply grounding remedy - akin to the tree remedies. At one point I felt like I was being pulled down into the ground. It was not unpleasant – in fact, il noticed it feeling good. Like a weighted blanket has been placed on me, weighing me to the ground.. I felt solid. Both my feet were planted firmly on the ground. I wanted to stomp, like a child singing *"The Grand old Duke of York"*, [a British nursery song where as little children we would stamp our feet when singing it]. I wanted to stamp my feet like a child - not throwing a tantrum, just wanting to feel the strength of my body pounding on the Earth. I felt a calling to be extra grounded.

Safety & Protection

I noticed feeling safe - and as though there was an invisible protective shield around me.

Manifestation & Materialisation

I was reminded of a teaching on manifestation & materialisation. I have always wished I knew where the original source of this teaching was from, so my apologies to the wise soul whose name I do not know, but whose teaching is, I feel, hugely important.

We talk a lot about manifestation, but when we look at the etymology of the word "manifestation", at its route is the word "man". It carries a masculine energy. When we look at the word "materialisation", at its route is the word "mater ". "Mater" is the Latin for "mother". This is what mothers do - they literally turn something that is envisioned as a wish or a dream into physical matter in the form of a child. To "materialise" is literally to turn something into physical reality - to mother or birth an idea into existence. "Mater" is similar to "Matter" - mothers turn their vision into *matter.* However, if we don't believe we matter, we cannot mater effectively either. Materialisation is to the feminine what manifestation is to the masculine.

This remedy reminds us of our power to make our dreams a reality - in alignment with whether we are going to be manifesting or materialising based on the alignment of our gender.

Structure

The structure itself is very important for stability. This means getting all the angles right, for optimal stability, and the structure being aligned for strength and longevity. There is a connection here with the correct proportions needed to ensure a perfect structure - and with that, stability and protection. I found myself thinking about mathematics, angles, engineers, architects.

This remedy may well be one that would support the work of architects and engineers in working on the most stable structures. Inherent in this is also an appreciation of angles we find in the natural world, including Phi mathematics and the proportions of the Golden Spiral. There is, in fact, a branch of architecture that is specifically aligned with Phi mathematics (and so ensuring the vibration of love flows freely throughout the spaces that are designed). It is called Phi architecture.

Community

Homes are places where loved ones gather. I had a strong sense with this remedy of community, connection, sharing, togetherness. A home, or a building, is a structure that facilitates gatherings. I was reminded of my times visiting my grandmother as a child, and she and her neighbours had an open door policy. I loved it. People would come in and out of each other's houses. A home wasn't a closed off box, like it is today. Home is supposed to be a place that shelters everyone from the weather, but in which food is prepared and made with love, to be shared with laughter, fun and joy.

I was reminded of how people would use their homes as places of religious worship during times of oppression. They are important places for communities together.

Warmth & Contentment

When love flows freely (Phi), and there is a sense of stability, safety, and community, then there is also the experience of warmth. It's interesting to me to look at a cube, which looks like it would have no warmth to it at all and yet I felt so much love, warmth and contentment when I thought about my family, and my son, sitting with this remedy. I felt contentment in my role as a mother too - and a sense of completion, as though my job has largely been done, in a nice way.

Mental / Emotional Symptoms

Homesick
Homelessness
Community - lack of
Community - desire for
Rootlessness
Uncertain of what home is and where to find it
Lack of care for the home
Hoarding

Dislike of cleaning
Loneliness
Ungrounded
Lost - feeling lost, cut adrift
Difficult to put roots down
Moves frequently
Home feels unsafe - currently or in the past
Feeling unsafe generally
Feeling trapped in a home that isn't nurturing or safe
Feeling of not mattering
Difficulties asking to have needs met

Physical Particular Symptoms

Head

Blows to the head
Cracked skull

Nose

Collapsed septum

Mouth & Teeth

Misaligned teeth

Throat

Difficulties asking to have needs met

Lungs & Breathing

Collapsed lung

Heart

Weak heart beat

Digestion

Constipation
Incomplete evacuation
Poor peristalsis

Female Reproductive

Structural issues with reproduction affecting fertility

Male Reproduction

Structural issues with reproduction affecting fertility

Back & Limbs

Stiffness in joints
Slowness in movements
Rheumatoid Arthritis
Stiffness, does not improve with movement
Osteoporosis
All musculoskeletal conditions

Physical General Symptoms

Sleep

Broken sleep
Light sleeper - does not drop into a deep sleep easily

Food & Drink

Desires staple foods - potatoes, root vegetables, may desire meat.
Better for these.
Dislike of fish and seafoods - these aggravate.
Thirstless

Energy Level

Slow, steady energy, similar to Calc carb

Clinical

Rheumatoid Arthritis
Osteoporosis
Fractures, broken bones
Sprains
Strains
All musculoskeletal conditions

Spiritual

"Home is where the heart is"

Remedy Affinities

Arnica
Bryonia
Calc carb
Calc phos
Magnesia muriatica
Oak

Petrified sequoia
Pulsatilla
Silver birch
Sulphur
Tabernanthe iboga (Declan Hammond)
Vernix caseosa
9/11 Survivor Tree

Octahedron

18 December 2025
East Sussex
England

This remedy was triturated from an essence prepared by the author using the intuitive trituration method. The substance was triturated to 13c in October 2025, with a follow-up proving conducted on 18 December 2025.

Triturated and proved by the author.

Octahedron

An octahedron is an eight-sided shape, made of eight equilateral triangles - it looks like two pyramids, with the bases glued together, and one pyramid pointing up, the other pointing down, forming a diamond shape. This symbolises Heaven and Earth meeting. It represents the element of Air.

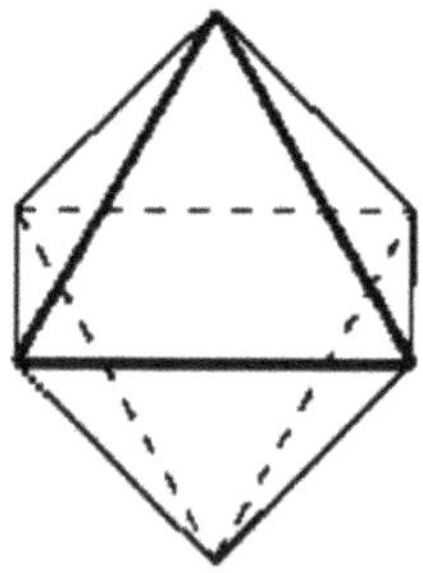

The octahedron represents balance, clarity, intellect, communication, and integration. It has a cerebral quality to it, and emphasises a strong connection with higher knowledge, and embodies truth, and compassion.

Octahedron Homeopathic Remedy™

Key Themes

Balance of knowledge, wisdom and feeling
Clarity of thought
Decision-making
Manifestation / Materialisation
Nervous system health
Microbiome & cellular consciousness
Detoxification
The anchoring of Light in the body
Healing & repairing the skin
Happiness

Balance of knowledge, wisdom and feeling

The octahedron represents accessing higher knowledge, and integrating it into the physical body and physical reality. It is the integration of spiritual understanding and physical matter.

One of the interfaces where we see the spiritual aspects of our existence meeting the physical matter of our bodies is where the endocrine system meets the chakra system.

To live in balance is to live in alignment with the fact that we are spiritual beings having a human experience, a Stephen Covey famously said. There is a higher knowledge, and a higher wisdom that we can connect with, and that is what the upper part of the octahedron connects us with. It is then anchored down and grounded into our existence on earth.

I was aware of all this knowledge, all these thoughts coming to me. The thoughts were very clear. Logical. But not clinical. The thoughts that came felt straightforward and practical, so that I could easily apply them in my life. They were clear and simple ideas and thoughts I could easily follow.

I was also aware of seeing each chakra spinning as though it were a diamond.

Clarity of thought

There is clarity of thought, and a directness of thinking in this remedy. Like a diamond cuts through the hardest natural materials on Earth, this remedy cuts through clouded thinking and uncertainty. There is a precision to thought. Laser sharp, and focused.

There is so much clarity in this remedy. Clear thought. It comes easily, smoothly.

Decision-making

Decision-making feels easier. Where there might be uncertainty, or anxiety about which decision feels most resonant, the clarity of thought this remedy brings also helps with decision making.

I don't love making decisions usually, but I found myself feeling more confident than usual with less worry over making the "right decision" in a particular context. It felt like the decision was clear - the choice stood above other options, almost like there was an arrow pointing towards it. It felt like I could easily make the decision and move on.

Manifestation / Materialisation

There is an "as above, so below" aspect to this remedy. I feel this is a remedy that very much is a bridge and connects what Archangels Metatron and Sandalphon represent.

These two Archangels are said to be the only ones that have truly lived on the Earth and had a human experience; as the twin sons of Abraham - Enoch and Elijah. Archangel Metatron is said to have been Enoch, and Archangel Sandalphon Elijah. Archangel Metatron represents healing systems and spiritual knowledge, Archangel Sandalphon represents grounding - including of that knowledge into the Earth and into our earthly existence.

There is an aspect of them both that therefore connects with manifestation and materialisation - bringing what our dreams in the heavens are (Archangel Metatron) down onto the Earth (Archangel Sandalphon).

I had a strong sense of this remedy acting like a prism through which higher frequencies come in and become focused into a single point. I imagine that I could take a pencil and write down all my desires on a piece of paper and the very desires would be able come down through the pencil to the very point with which I was writing; the point of the pencil that meets the paper I would write on. It is as though the energy of my wishes and dreams could be harnessed into that singular point and the possibility for it to exist.

I could also see diamonds that were sparkly and shiny. I felt an abundance in this remedy. There was a sense of wealth associated with it- bringing through from the heavens what is needed.

Nervous system health

I experienced a strong connection with the nervous system through this remedy, in particular the myelin sheath and cerebrospinal fluid. I kept experiencing the winding of the myelin sheath as it is laid down, it feels like this remedy gives a solidity to it.

I had a sense of the speed of the information travelling across neural networks, jumping rapidly between the nodes of Ranvier (natural gaps in the myelin sheath that speed up the travel of electrical impulses). I sensed the movement of the electrical impulses as feeling rapid, unimpeded, vibrant, alive. It felt like there are no obstacles anywhere, the electrical impulses flowed freely and smoothly.

Microbiome & cellular consciousness

I also had a sense of how much the microbiome loves this remedy. It powers it up, bridging any gaps, connecting the different aspects that make it up. Light. There is so much Light in this remedy. It dispels darkness, and stagnation and sluggishness, so that it can be expelled.

This is a remedy that speaks to the T-junctions in the gut, tightening them. Like a laser light being used along a loose junction to tighten it, the downward point of the octahedron can harness the healing of the cosmos and harness it down to the physical.

Detoxification

This is a remedy that supports detoxification - I had a sense of how it anchors in light to what has become stuck, and then spins through it to break it down so it can be expelled safely.

Almost as though a drill is drilling through the stuck, solid masses and areas, blasting through and breaking it down.

This remedy is supportive of the liver.

The anchoring of Light in the body - vitamin D3 pathways, water & mitochondria

There is so much Light in this remedy. Huge amounts of Light. This is a remedy that anchors Light in the body. It is involved in vitamin D3 and how it anchors light into the body.

This is a remedy that also supports mitochondrial health. Whereas the Golden Spiral speaks to the spirals within the mitochondria, this remedy speaks to the whole mitochondria as an organelle that converts light into energy.

Healing & repairing the skin

This remedy can help bring healing and repair to the skin. Where there is redness, it can soothe. Where is rawness and burning it can calm. Where the skin needs to be repaired, in a smilier way to how the point of the octahedron can repair T junctions, it can also repair breaks in the skin.

Happiness

There is happiness in this remedy - a lightness, and a happiness - like the sun reflected on water on a comfortably warm day. There is a contentedness in this remedy; a feeling of having everything we need.

Mental / Emotional Symptoms

Difficulties making decisions
Indecisiveness
Uncertain of decisions
Fear of making mistakes
Lack of confidence
Lack of self-belief
Fogginess in thought
Lack of clarity of thought
Lack
Feeling of poverty
Feeling of not having enough
Disgruntled
Sadness
Disappointment with life

Physical Particular Symptoms

Head

Confusion
Brain fog

Eyes

Poor vision
Difficulties seeing
Cataracts
Astigmatism

Ears

Sensitive hearing
Difficulties hearing

Nose

Congestion
Loss of smell

Throat

Tonsillitis

Lungs & Breathing

Pneumonia
Bronchitis
Toxicity accumulated in lungs

Heart

Irregular heartbeat
Heart palpitations

Digestion

Dysbiosis

Crohn's disease
Leaky gut
Sluggish bowel
Build up of old faecal matter in colon walls

Liver

Supports the work of the liver lobules
Cholestasis
Sluggish liver

Kidneys

Chronic Kidney Disease

Bladder

Cloudy urine

Female Reproductive

Blocked fallopian tubes

Male Reproduction

Blocked tubes

Back & Limbs

Muscular tears

Skin

Redness

Red rash
Urticaria
Wounds - open skin

Physical General Symptoms

Food & Drink

Thirsty - needs plenty of water
Desire for salads
Desire for foods containing water eg fruits

Energy Level

Slow, steady energy, similar to Calc carb

Clinical

Mitochondrial issues
Immune system difficulties
Cataracts
Dysbiosis
Leaky gut
Anaemia
Irregular heartbeat
Palpitations
Fungal toe nails
Sluggish liver
Cholestasis
Chronic Kidney Disease

Spiritual

Facilitates manifestation / materialisation

Ungrounded

Remedy Affinities

Aurum
Baryta carb
Cann-i
Diamond
Golden Spiral
Graphites
Lycopodium
Metatron's Cube
Milky Way
Okoubaka
Onosmodium
Petrified Sequoia
Pulsatilla

Icosahedron

19 December 2025
East Sussex
England

This remedy was triturated from an essence prepared by the author using the intuitive trituration method. The substance was triturated to 13c in October 2025, with a follow-up proving conducted on 19 December 2025.

Triturated and proved by the author.

Icosahedron

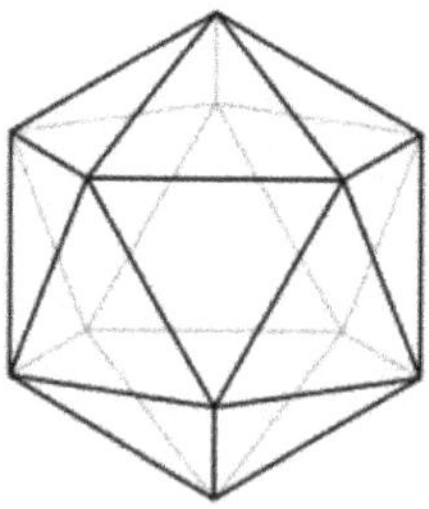

An icosahedron is a twenty-sided shape, made of twenty equilateral triangles.

The icosahedron is associated with the element of water which is fluid, and connects us with flow, with our emotions, and being able to express them. It is also linked to the sacral chakra and our ability express our emotions, particularly in relationship with others. Emotional healing and transformation are also represented with this Platonic Solid.

Our emotions connect us with our intuition, so there is an intuitive aspect to this icosahedrons.

Icosahedron Homeopathic Remedy™

Key Themes

Instability to Stability
Revealing & Healing the Hidden Inner Child
Visibility / Being seen
Authenticity & Joy
Childlike Wonder
Play
Mitochondria & the Microbiome

Instability to Stability

This remedy has themes of stability, and changeability. Both when trituration the remedy and then later proving once more, I felt really wobbly. I hadn't remembered which of the Platonic solids had made me feel this during the December proving, and this was really interesting to me to see this repeated once I realised it was the same. I felt unstable, like I couldn't find my footing. It was quite disconcerting. I felt I had nothing to hold on to, and like I could have just rolled away, which felt uncomfortable. It also gave me a sense of feeling quite alone, and on my own, with nothing to support me. I was aware of having to deal with the wobbliness on my own.

Revealing & Healing the Hidden Inner Child

This remedy brought up a feeling of being alone with the physical wobble, which triggered uncomfortable feelings. This is a remedy that can reveal the inner child. I was aware of a large mirror in the room I was in, I felt it was necessary to feel the discomfort and allow it to flow and move out before being able to return to steadiness. There was a need to hold on to something, but there was nothing to hold on to, which brought up a desire to cry like a child. This remedy is one that can help those who need a good cry to release some sadness, sorrow and deep grief. On the other side of the release is lightness. There is a deep transformation in this remedy - a releasing of a lot of emotion, a deep healing, that doesn't have to be protracted. Perhaps because of working at a sacred geometry / soul level, it felt that even five minutes of crying, would release 20 minutes' worth of crying under normal circumstances The release of emotions is speeded up, like a turbo transformation of stuck emotion.

I was reminded of little children when they throw a tantrum. They are so real, honest and raw as they throw themselves on the ground and pump with their little fists and their little kicking feet. They are true, and authentic, and there is something so beautiful about seeing such honest expressions of emotion, that we just don't express as adults. I'm sure all of us at times if we were allowed, have some inner child part of us that would probably wish to throw ourselves down on the ground and stamp and pummel it all out like little children do. We lose the ability to be so honest with our emotions as we grow. This remedy connects us with our honest emotions, free from shame or judgement, with an "Ah! Hello! There you are, I see you. I recognise you are a part of me, and I can hold you, and love you and accept you.". There is a liberation in this remedy. It doesn't feel like a painful or difficult experience, just honest and revealing and healing – we don't have to go through the whole experience of feeling everything that we carry. It's merely an invitation for recognition. Honouring. Like how a light particle vanishes when looked it, this is the same. This is for the emotions we have stuffed away and not acknowledged. They don't need to be fully felt, just seen and acknowledged. This remedy merely allows that stuck hidden inner child emotion to be seen and acknowledged before it is transformed. This goes to the depths of our hidden inner child. There is so much lightness at the end of this. Freedom. And then the wobbliness transforms into being able to move with joy, and happiness like a child dancing, leaping from left foot to right foot waving their arms in the air with delight. The wobbliness becomes joy, freedom to play, roll around, move about, flow, be unconstrained happiness.

Visibility / Being seen

As this is a remedy that reveals hidden emotions, it makes sense that this is a remedy about visibility – what is seen, and what is unseen. What we are comfortable revealing, of ourselves. Have we been hiding ourselves away, with fear, guilt or shame? Are we willing to let this go, and step out into the light and be seen for all that we are?

Authenticity & Joy

There is an authenticity to this remedy. This remedy celebrates our authentic selves. It sets us free to connect with our true essence, the expression of our personality, our joy. Every child arrives with joy. Life may squash that out of us, but we arrive with joy. This is a remedy to take us back to that joy, the essence of our soul. To be who we really are, beyond all the layers of who we have been told we should be.

This remedy carries the vibration of the younger generations, who are more free, authentic, expressive.

Childlike Wonder

This remedy moves us out of the stories we tell ourselves, and the thinking that goes on in our head, and into being embodied, more present in the moment.

One there had been some healing for the inner child, there was just a desire to play and have fun. The stories just didn't matter. There was a desire to experience joy and happiness once more. Play on swings. It was close to Christmas when this was proved,, and I was reminded of the scene in the film *Elf*, where Will Ferrell's Elf character makes himself some food in the home of his Dad. He makes a bowl of pasta, covers it with sweets (candies), and syrup, breaks up a chocolate pop tart and then mushes it all together with his hands, before eating it with his hands. This is a remedy that has that energy to it. Having lots of unadulterated fun. I mean even that word – unadulterated – it literally means without having put all that adult thinking on top. A childlike wonder and joy. This is a remedy for the inner child - for when we've become too serious, are carrying a lot of responsibilities, when adulting has taken over our lives. This is a remedy to remind us to play. Surely that's why we came [to Earth]? To play at being human, to experience, to remember the good times, and that they are possible. Even though life can be tough sometimes, we can still find time to play as children do?

Play

Inherent in this remedy is the vibration of play. We can't get to the joy and childlike wonder if we have any deeply buried suppressed emotions. So this remedy helps clear some of that so that we can connect with our inner child and play. This is how the remedy raises our vibration - it connects us with joyful fun and play once some of what is stuck gets released.

Mitochondria & the Microbiome

There is such a strong feeling with this remedy that the

mitochondria and microbiome love this remedy, It literally anchors in light! Joy happiness! Like children skipping along merrily together. It brings in collective happiness and joy that is also felt as a cellular and ecosystem level in the body.

Mental / Emotional Symptoms

Too much adulting
Too serious
Lack of joy
Lack of happiness
Deeply stuck and suppressed emotions
Fear of expressing emotions
Hidden emotions
Hiding self
Fear of being seen
Reluctance to sing or dance
Forgotten how to have fun
Lost inner child
Feeling the weight of too many responsibilities
Lack of authenticity
Disconnection from self
Doesn't know how to be themselves
Attached to stories in their lives
Overthinking
Too much in the head and not in the body
Future planning
Always thinking ahead
Not in the present moment
Needing lightness, laughter
Says "doesn't care" about relationships, as a reason to have plenty of sex with many partners, but deep down is yearning to be held and loved

Physical Particular Symptoms

Head

Overthinking
Fuzzy feeling at top of head

Eyes

Sore eyes
Eyes sore from crying
Tired eyes
Dust in the eyes
Red eyes from chlorinated pool

Ears

Sensitive hearing

Mouth & Teeth

Cavities

Lungs & Breathing

Alveoli
Poor gaseous exchange at alveoli
Opens air sacs to receive oxygen

Heart

Bradycardia
Prolongation of diastole

Digestion

Dysbiosis
Sluggish bowel
Build up of old faecal matter in colon walls

Bladder

Acidic urine
Strong smelling urine
Dark yellow urine
Turbid urine

Female Reproductive

Dark blood in menses
Clots

Male Reproduction

Focus on sex rather than making love
Lack of intimacy in sexual experiences
Fear of intimacy in sexual experiences

Back & Limbs

Stiffness due to lack of movement

Skin

Keratosis pilaris
Cradle cap

Physical General Symptoms

Dreams

Dreams of falling
Dreams of buildings collapsing

Food & Drink

Desire for cheese and dairy

Clinical

Mitochondrial issues
Dysbiosis
Leaky gut
Bradycardia
Adrenal fatigue
Chronic fatigue syndrome
Keratosis pilaris
Cradle cap

Spiritual

Healing of inner child
Expression of inner child
Reconnection with joy and happiness

Remedy Affinities

Apple Tree
Arsenicum
Aurum met
Aurum mur
Ayahuasca
Banyan Tree (Guild)
Frankincense
Nat carb
Nat mur
Sepia
Silver birch
Thuja
Thymus gland

Dodecahedron

20 December 2025
East Sussex
England

This remedy was triturated from an essence prepared by the author using the intuitive trituration method. The substance was triturated to 13c in October 2025, with a follow-up proving conducted on 20 December 2025.

Triturated and proved by the author.

Dodecahedron

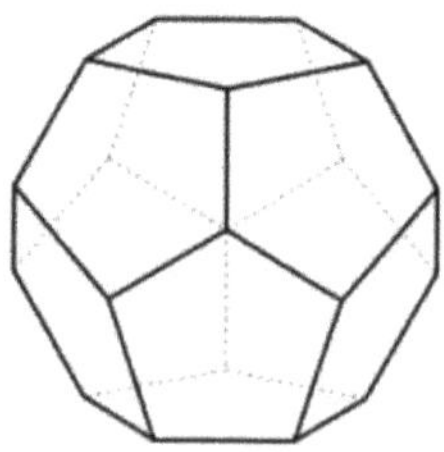

A dodecahedron is a twelve-sided shape, made of twelve pentagons. Pentagons are a clear expression of Phi mathematics, with the ratio of the length of a diagonal to the length of a side being exactly 1.618. We can see how the Golden Spiral directly connects with the pentagon in the diagram below. There is also the "Golden Hexagram", which demonstrates how the Milky Way emerges - a flow of spirals, but if you look close up at edges, they are actually lines; the masculine holding the flow of the feminine.

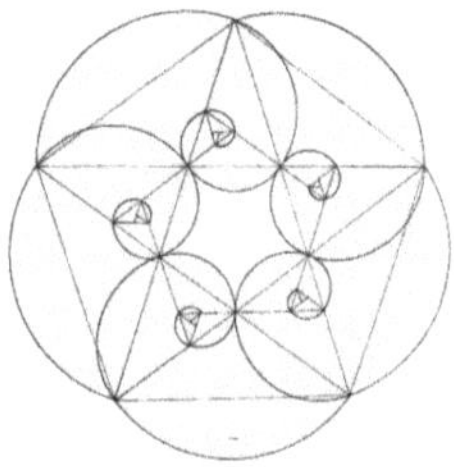

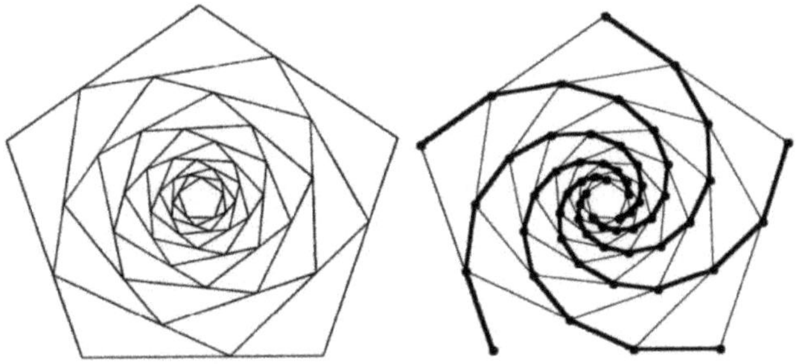

As we can see here from these Fibonacci / Golden Pentagons, this is how we see the spiral emerge in the plant kingdom' in the unfolding of roses, and cabbages. I wonder if it could be a doctrine of signature of the unfolding patterns of the Universe.

The pentagon is a true expression of the vibration of love. 12 pentagons together forming a dodecahedron is said to an expression of the structure of the Universe.

The number 12 represents Divine order, perfection in that order, completeness, wholeness. 12 is an important number numerological in it's own right, and then it becomes 3 when the 1+2 are added together using Pythagorean numerology. The number 3 represents integration - the coming together of the body, mind and spirit, or Father, Son and Holy Ghost. So there is another layer to the wholeness and completeness that the 12 pentagons bring. We see 12 a lot in spiritual meanings - for example in 12 signs of the Western Astrological Zodiac, or the 12 disciples of Jesus that are taught (although there were more, and an equal number of women disciples too).

The dodecahedron is associated with the element of aether, or spirit, and is said to connect us with the Universe and with Source, or the Divine. So this is a Platonic solid that helps us to connect with a much greater, more expanded awareness of the true nature of reality. As we are connecting with the vibration of Source energy, the depths of the healing transcends all time and space, so works with us in a multidimensional way. The dodecahedron helps us to connect with our guardian angels and spirit guides, as well as our loved ones in spirit. As already mentioned, the dodecahedron is considered by some to be the expression of the structure of the Universe.

Dodecahedron Homeopathic Remedy™

Key Themes

Balance & Fairness
Compassion
Healing
Feeling supported when feeling alone
Multidimensionality
Compassion
Sovereignty
Structures that support life

Balance & Fairness

The Scales of Justice are an important aspect of this remedy. The Scales of Justice, in their truest form, are about balance, fairness, and a restoration of that balance and fairness where this has been lost. Fairness is a central theme to this remedy. Where we have extended too far into polarity states, this brings us back to balance. Where Vector Equilibrium brings us from duality to unity in the centre, dodecahedron behaves in a similar way - however has the additional vibration of being held by Source as this happens. And so there is an extra layer of comfort in this remedy as the nervous system regulates in a deeper, and more held way. The Scales of Justice can hold different perspectives at the same time, and this is reflected in this remedy. Almost like a kindly, loving parent can hold the different emotional states of a child with love and grace and support, dodecahedron can hold different perspectives and states lovingly, without judgement, just coming to a place of balance and fairness. Vector equilibrium seeks to move from duality to centre, collapsing the different extremes and returning to centre. Whereas dodecahedron holds all of the perspectives lovingly, in a way that eases any tension between them.

Compassion

Inherent within being able to hold balance and fairness, especially in difficult circumstances is compassion. When sitting with this remedy, I was really taken back to having seen the film *I Swear,* a remarkable film telling the deeply profound story of John Davidson, who bravely brought to bring to the world an understanding of Tourette's syndrome. A very humble man from Scotland, he sought to educate people about it through his own experience as someone with Tourette's syndrome who was completely misunderstood - at times dangerously so - because people didn't know about Tourette's syndrome when he was young. It's one of the most powerful films I've ever seen. I was lucky enough to watch it in a cinema that was packed, and I think everybody at some point in the cinema was crying like a baby, and at other times roaring with laughter. And yet the main thread through this film is an incredible, deep feeling of compassion for what John has walked through. It is a film that draws out compassion for our fellow humans in a way that is deep, and heartfelt, and truly human - loving our fellow humans, seeing them with their pain and struggles, and wishing for them to know peace, support, understanding, love. What John Davidson has achieved is remarkable.

This remedy, I feel, connects us with the deepest aspects of compassion for one another. Perhaps this is because this remedy connects us with Source; Divinity; transcending the divisions that we can experience with one another as humans. As homeopaths we aim to practice as Dr Hahnemann said as "unprejudiced observers". This is very much a remedy that takes us to the vibration that Dr Hahnemann wished for us to practice with.

Even if some relationships are too harmful to be a part of, and we have to maintain healthy boundaries for our well-being, this remedy brings a deep compassion for those that may have caused us pain.

Healing

This remedy brings deep healing, through Source. It regulates the nervous system, and helps us to feel held.

Feeling supported when feeling alone

The dodecahedron connects us with spirit. This means with our loved ones in spirit, our guardian angels, and our spirit guides. This may be a useful remedy for those who feel alone, forsaken, abandoned, unsupported. I am reminded of the poem Footsteps In The Sand by Mary Stevenson.

"One night I dreamed I was walking along the beach with the Lord.
Many scenes from my life flashed across the sky.In each scene I
noticed footprints in the sand.Sometimes there were two sets of
footprints,other times there were one set of footprints.

This bothered me because I noticedthat during the low periods of
my life,when I was suffering fromanguish, sorrow or defeat,

I could see only one set of footprints.
So I said to the Lord,"You promised me Lord,that if I followed you,you would walk with me always.
But I have noticed that duringthe most trying periods of my lifethere have only been oneset of footprints in the sand.Why, when I needed you most,you have not been there for me?"

The Lord replied,"The times when you haveseen only one set of footprints,is when I carried you."

Mary Stevenson

This is a remedy that connects us with this feeling of being carried for those that feel alone.

Multidimensionality

This is a remedy that transcends time and space. The dodecahedron is said to be the structure of the Universe. Many realities exist within it. This is a remedy that holds all existence simultaneously in balance - just as the many different perspectives and states are held as we explored in the key theme of Balance & Fairness, this is a remedy that speaks to all experiences across time and space.

Sovereignty

As the dodecahedron ensures there is space for everything within it, it means that there is space for everyone within it. Everyone to be truly who they are – and that means to be sovereign. All of the sacred geometry remedies speak to sovereignty. Dodecahedron speaks to being seen as a sovereign being by others as well as seeing oneself as being sovereign.

This remedy speaks to the spirit in Goethe's terms, the super ego in Freud's terms, God or source in others. This remedy is about being witnessed by Divinity; fully seen and accepted.

In sitting with this remedy, I reflect upon how patriarchal structures seek to ensure that we are not seen; we become invisible. In the process, we lose our connection to our sovereignty. Being seen, witnessed as existing, and mattering is hugely important. Indigenous peoples the world over have had to endure attempts to wipe out their existence. Or simply being ignored by settlers. So much work is being done to try to address this around the world but it is important to note that this is a feature of this remedy.

We are *seen* by Source, therefore we *exist.* Therefore we *matter.* Therefore we are *sovereign.*

Structures that support life

There is an enduring quality to this remedy. It connects us with the structures that we need to have in place that support life. Those structures being present with grace and ease. The structures include the natural world, plants, the nourishment within biodynamic soils and the foods grown with care and love for the Earth.

I have been reminded of the old boiler, in the house where I live, which is about 40 or 45 years old. It is mechanical, with few electrical parts, and so just keeps on going. It is built for durability. The gas engineers who come and service it are all younger than the age of the boiler, and they always get really excited to see it. It's like a museum relic. But it was built with durability in mind. Not making money through constant upgrades, and not according to planned obsolescence. This remedy speaks to the structures that exist out of care for who and what they are supporting, rather than care for self at the expense of others.

That is the state of nature. The natural world provides generously, reliably, with durability without enslaving us to keep returning beyond its natural lifespan.

This is a remedy that helps us respect the natural structures in the world, whilst also helping us discern which of the modern structures are necessary to support our lives. There is a little less need for material goods that are disposable inherent in this remedy.

Mental / Emotional Symptoms

Alone
Lonely
Foresaken
Abandoned
Unsupported
Lack of fairness
Not being seen by those who matter
Invisible
Not being validated
Lack of power
Lack of sovereignty
Lack of balance
Facing or feeling injustice(s)
Lack of compassion
In need of compassion
Lack of empathy
Everything feels too much
Materialism out of balance
Orphans
Difficulties making decisions

Physical Particular Symptoms

Head

Throbbing headache - left temple
Throbbing headache - left above the eye
Throbbing headache - left side extending to throbbing pain in left eye

Eyes

Loss of vision - left eye
Blurry vision - left eye

Ears

Eustacian tube - sensation of trickle down eustachian tube
Gentle throbbing - left ear

Nose

Coryza - fluid, clear, copious
Sneezing - caused by dust
Sneezing - during cold

Mouth & Teeth

Halitosis

Throat

Swollen glands
Difficulty swallowing

Lungs & Breathing

Difficulties opening lungs fully to inhale full amount of air
Constricted breathing
Laboured breathing
Wheezing worse hot, dry weather
Wheezing worse humidity

Heart

Cardiomyopathy
Slow heart beat
Irregular heart beat
Angina

Digestion

Dysbiosis
Crohns's disease
Coeliac disease
Inflammatory bowel disease
Irritable bowel syndrome

Liver & Gallbladder

Liver toxicity
Cirrhosis

Bladder

Frequency of urination
Nocturia
Burning when peeing
Cystitis
Female Reproductive System

Imbalanced hormones

Back & Limbs

Osteoporosis

Skin

Acne vulgaris
Acne rosacea

Physical General Symptoms

Sleep

Insomnia
Difficulties falling asleep
Lies awake for a long time
Shallow sleep - does not sleep deeply for long
Restless sleep
Disturbed sleep

Dreams

Dreams of ghosts
Dreams of monsters
Dreams of keys - either held in the hand or lost keys
Dreams of roses - being given roses
Dreams of walking in rose garden
Dreams of being able to smell the scent of a rose
Dreams of robins

Food & Drink

Desire for alcohol
Alcohol agg
Meat agg
Dairy agg

Energy

May present like Calc carb - slow and steady

Clinical

Cardiomyopathy
Crohns's disease
Coeliac disease
Inflammatory bowel disease
Irritable bowel syndrome
Cirrhosis
Cystitis
Osteoporosis
Autoimmune conditions

Spiritual

Scales of Justice
Fairness
Balance
Compassion
Forsaken - welcomes feeling of support

Remedy Affinities

Aconite
Buddleja
All the Lac remedies
Calc carb
Calc phos
Chamomilla
Green
Holly
Medorrhinum
Nettle (Guild)
Phos
Pulsatilla
Yellow

Prescribing Notes

1) This remedy is very similar to Calc carb - there may be a slowness and steadiness in the person. They may take their time to make decisions.

Metatron's Cube

29 October 2025
East Sussex
England

This remedy was triturated from an essence prepared by the author using the intuitive trituration method. The substance was triturated to 13c in October 2025, with a follow-up proving that was conducted on 29 October 2025 at the Golden Spiral International School of Homeopathy™ with students and teachers joining from around the world.

Metatron's Cube

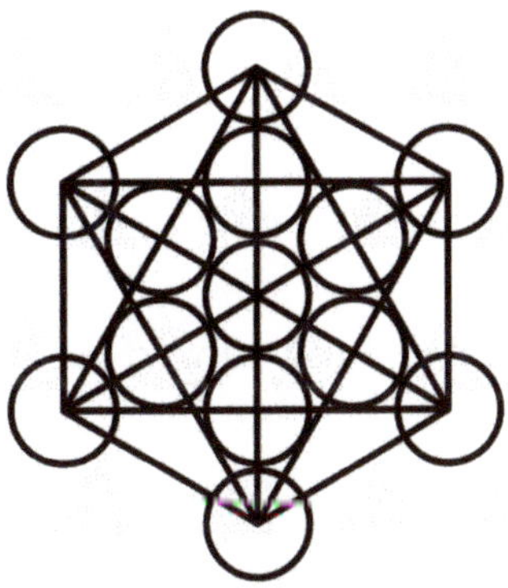

Metatron's Cube is not itself a Platonic solid - or a polygon. It is a sacred symbol into which all of the Platonic solids can be embedded.

It is said to be representation of Archangel Metatron, the Archangel of all healing systems and knowledge of healing and medicine. Archangel Metatron is to have been the guide for Dr Mikao Usui to receive the Reiki symbols.

I believe Archangel Metatron to be the true Source of homeopathy knowledge - and that he was guiding Dr Hahnemann's discoveries. Metatron's Cube is a symbol that takes us to the blueprint of creation. Lines are drawn to connect all of the circles found in the Fruit of Life.

Metatron's Cube Homeopathic Remedy™

Key Themes

Event Horizon - centre of all creation in the Universe
Vortexes
Possibilities
Infinite Abundance
Ecstasy, Joy & Bliss
Reset & Birth
Collapsing timelines
Clearing trauma
Clearing all that isn't in alignment
Amma
Spirals within spirals - the Mandelbrot Set
Connection with Nature
Stepping into Service & Life Purpose

Event Horizon - centre of all creation in the Universe

When I made this remedy, it is not an exaggeration to say that I had one of the most amazing experiences of my life. I experienced travelling to the Event Horizon - the very centre of the Universe from which everything emerges. I had no fear, just pure joy; true bliss. I knew whilst there that I could request anything and I could call it forth from the Event Horizon. I felt so happy there, it was total ecstasy.

I was at the threshold where all possibility is accessible and it felt infinitely remarkable. I felt a joy, happiness and delight coursing through every part of my being that I felt only a tiny handful of times in my life. It was pure bliss.

I felt like my life on Earth was very far away - that any earthly worries and cares were very far away too. I felt like I was in the centre of all Creation, and like I could float in it, calling forth whatever I chose.

I was travelling through wormholes, past black holes. I felt like I was experiencing all time and space, and I could move fast through time and space and the "past" was collapsing.

It opens up the possibility of ancestors also experiencing what we experience. he sacred geometry remedies don't just work on us, they work on our nearest ancestors when we take them - like the degrees of influence, that the remedies travel back through the generations.

Vortexes

Several provers described experienced entering a vortex.

Sunlight structures water - it turns H_2O (unstructured water) into structured H_3O_2 water - hexagonal lattices that Professor Gerald Pollack has measured, and calls the 4th phase of water - or Exclusion Zone (EZ) water. It's incredible - it's how water becomes geometric, and so can carry electrical charge and light.

A vortex can also structure water - and an energy vortex in the air structures the light energy; photons, and the air to do the same thing - to become geometric; in other words to carry electrical charge, light and energy.

Vortexes amplify our connections with each other, with love, with consciousness, with nature, and help us to discharge stress and difficult nervous system (electrical) energy, so that our nervous systems can regulate. They can help us re-centre when we have become fragmented.

Many provers described feeling tingling, which also is an alignment with energy.

Possibilities

There is an opening up to new possibilities with this remedy. Some provers made some important new decisions in their lives.

One prover shared her experience of connecting with the possibility of love.

"I experienced this feeling of being in a vortex and I could see this man coming towards me, trying to grab my hand. I was trying to move towards him and I was trying to grab his hand and things were spinning and spinning and I felt like I really needed to grab his hand. We were spinning towards each other.

I have dreamt of this man a few times [in the last few months]. It's the same man and we were trying to catch each other in this space. It felt very real and I could see the colour of his skin and hair and the shirt was red and checked.......to experience that sensation and feeling and grab his hand would of course be amazing!".

Infinite Abundance

In this place of joy and bliss, I felt there was little materially that I wanted to call in, as I realised that I was content with what I have. I felt a total love for nature, and trees, and the seas, and the beautiful animal kingdom, and all I wanted was for everyone and everything on Earth to be happy and at peace.

I really felt how infinite abundance is - how in me reaching for my desires doesn't deprive anyone else of theirs. And I just knew and felt deeply in my core that it was my Divine right to receive all my dreams and wishes. Any anxieties, any worries - simply didn't -

couldn't - exist in this place. I really felt how I am a soul that is worthy of all the wonderful things I wish for. I

I could see all of the beautiful woven invisible bonds that connect all planets in the solar system, the organs in our bodies. I could see all of the bonds as light energy bridges; a beautiful interconnected web of light travelling, weaving, connecting.

Ecstasy, Joy & Bliss

I experienced a deep sense of profound ecstasy; the most heart-expanding bliss and joy imaginable. It was peaceful joy, not wild at all - completely transcendent.

This was also an experience shared with some other provers too.

Reset & Birth

I felt as though I had experienced a complete reset - mind, body and soul. It feels like a remedy that can clear much trauma. A doorway can open to new possibilities.

One prover described receiving great clarity around her next steps in life, and making some really big life decisions, that were very much a reset - and a clearing of what hadn't been in alignment.

There is a starting anew; afresh, free from the challenges of the past - the theme of birth is very much alive in this remedy.

Collapsing Timelines

There is the experience of completing cycles in this remedy - collapsing timelines - a true starting again.

Clearing trauma

I literally felt like I was being reborn out of joy. I feel this remedy resets us in a way that clears trauma. It's like it takes us back to the beginning of time - creation - and helps us to start again. It burns off so much trauma.

Clearing all that isn't in alignment

This remedy also clears away - literally transmutes that which isn't in alignment. It's like there is no room for anything that is not in alignment in order for us to live a life where we are fully realised, where our spirit and soul soar.

That may not be easy to process, but necessary if we are to share our greatest brightest selves. Anything that holds us back has to be cleared.

Amma

Soon after the making and proving of this reedy, I went to see Amma in London with a friend. I feel there is a strong connection with Amma and all she represents with this remedy. I am not an "Amma devotee" in the formal sense of the word, but I have seen Amma several times. She is said to be an Avatar. She sits for DAYS and hugs thousands and thousands of people - even still now, in her early 70s. One of the things that strikes me about Amma is how much good she does with all the money she raises. The millions of women and girls and people she has helped with setting up microeconomics in India, or ensuring education for girls and all those in poverty, or with disaster relief efforts, or with supporting natural farming practices, or with teaching women to become plumbers and builders so they can build beautiful, safe latrines, the state-of-the-art hospitals that have homeopathy integrated into them. She does more than anyone else I have heard of on the planet to truly make a difference to millions of people's lives - but we don't hear of her in the mainstream. She's an inspiration.

When I think of Amma, I feel she represents such a wonderful alignment with the Divine, with love. With community, connection. I also feel that there is an invitation to us to share our best selves, our greatest selves - to truly be in Service to love.

I feel this is a remedy that invites us to do this - to live in greater service to love. It is said that whereas our Guardian Angels support us in our individual journeys through life, the Archangels help us with our work in service to something much bigger - in ways that help Mama Gaia and all of life on Earth as well as humanity.

This very much feels as though it is a remedy that calls this in.

Spirals within spirals - the Mandelbrot Set

This is a remedy that takes us to the centre of the Mandelbrot set which I also describe in the Golden Spiral proving. This is the point at which chaos and order meet, and the fractals of spirals emerge. We need both chaos and order - and an equal balance of both - for the spiral to emerge and flow beautifully in flow. This is a remedy that takes us to that vibration of true balance. This vibration - like all vibrations - has a sound frequency attached to it, and this remedy expresses that.

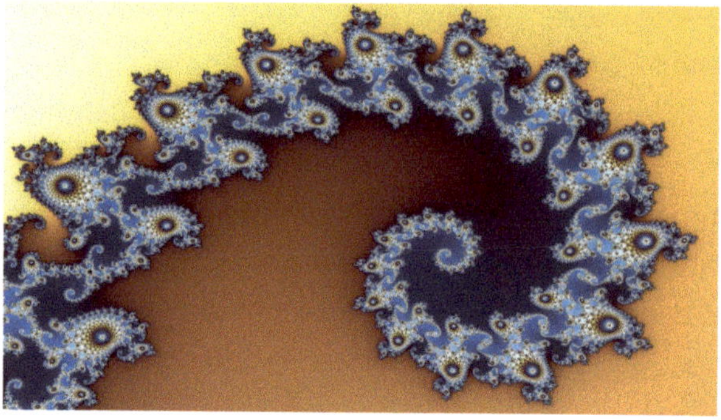

Connection with Nature

Several provers experienced animals appearing and coming close. When writing about this remedy, I had a ladybird come and walk all over my laptop, up and down the monitor, over the keys, over me, for over an hour, and would have continued had I not had to get up and go elsewhere.

Other provers saw a deer. Some became acutely aware of the sounds of animals, including one of an owl hooting. One who isn't usually keen on dogs found themselves feeling greater ease and appreciation for a dog that wanted to be with them than this person normally would be comfortable with.

Stepping into Service & Life Purpose

This is a remedy that connects us with what we are here to do in service, and helps us step away from what isn't in alignment with what we would do if we were in service.

The Archangels, as I have already shared, support us in our work in service, and this is what this remedy connects us with.

Marianne Williamson, in her beautiful book *The Law of Divine Compensation: On Work, Money and Miracles*[47], she shares deep wisdom on how many when seeking to earn more money will pray and ask "how can I make more money?" - when the question that really brings more money and abundance is "God, how can I best *serve*?"

This is a remedy that calls us to *service* for a more beautiful life and world for everyone. It transcends ego, and brings us to service in a way that is about the betterment of humanity and our beautiful planet, as well as the healing all our ancestors.

Mental / Emotional Symptoms

Ancestral trauma
Intergenerational trauma
Many obstacles in life
Cannot identify solutions to challenges
Feeling stuck
Lack of courage to do what needs to be done
Fear of next steps
Fear of change
Weighed down by problems
Weighed down by responsibilities

47 Marianne Williamson (2012) *The Law of Divine Compensation: On Work, Money and Miracles* HarperOne

Depression
Anxiety
Lack of joy
Unhappiness
Pessimism
Disconnection from life
Disconnection from loved ones
Disconnection from nature
Disconnection from spiritual aspect of self and life
Materialistic
Repeating same patterns
Not living ones life path or purpose
Lack of purpose
Addictions
Lack of power
Lack of sovereignty
Lack of flow in life
Energy attachments
Confusion
Difficult decision making
Grief
Lack of balance
Procrastination
Difficulties expressing needs & desires

Physical Particular Symptoms

Head

Adrenal headache
Pressure in the centre of the forehead
Tingling at the top of the head
Heavy head

Eyes

Macular degeneration
Whites of eyes yellow

Ears

Blocked ears
Build up of wax

Nose

Congested nose
Polylps

Mouth & Teeth

Tooth decay

Lungs & Breathing

Difficulties opening lungs fully to inhale full amount of air
Shallow breathing
Asthma

Heart

Poor circulation of blood

Digestion

Dysbiosis
Acidity
Crohns's disease
Coeliac disease
Inflammatory bowel disease
Irritable bowel syndrome
Polyps

Liver & Gallbladder

Liver toxicity
Cirrhosis
Fibrosis
Cholestasis

Bladder

Crystals in Urine

Female Reproductive System

Infertility
Birth

Male Reproductive System
Infertility

Back & Limbs

Osteoporosis
Degenerative conditions

Skin

Dermatitis

Physical General Symptoms

Dreams

Dreams of ancestors
Dreams of space
Dreams of the cosmos
Dreams of the stars

Food & Drink

Too many processed foods

Energy

Low energy
Restlessness
Moves from one extreme to the other

Clinical

Crohns's disease
Coeliac disease
Inflammatory bowel disease
Irritable bowel syndrome
Cirrhosis
Fibrosis
Cholestasis
Osteoporosis

Poor circulation
Autoimmune conditions

Spiritual

Ancestral trauma
Intergenerational trauma
Many obstacles in life
Cannot identify solutions to challenges
Feeling stuck
Lack of courage to do what needs to be done
Disconnection from life
Disconnection from loved ones
Disconnection from nature
Disconnection from spiritual aspect of self and life
Materialistic
Repeating same patterns
Not living ones life path or purpose
Lack of purpose

Remedy Affinities

Golden Spiral
Dodecahedron
Milky Way
Orange
Vector Equilibrium

Prescribing Notes

1) As I shared in the introduction, with all of the sacred geometry remedies, I recommend a potency of 30c - and I say that as someone who loves high potency remedies.

Except this one. IF someone's vital force can receive it well, this is the one remedy I would give in high potencies automatically. My favourite for this remedy is 50M. But if that is too high for some, then a 1M or 10M, but I really feel it's the 50M that welcomes in a full reset.

Part 4

Sacred Sites & Stars Aligned with the Golden Spiral

The Bosnian Pyramid of the Sun

16 March 2025
K2
Inside the tunnels of the Bosnian Pyramid of the Sun
Visoko
Bosnia

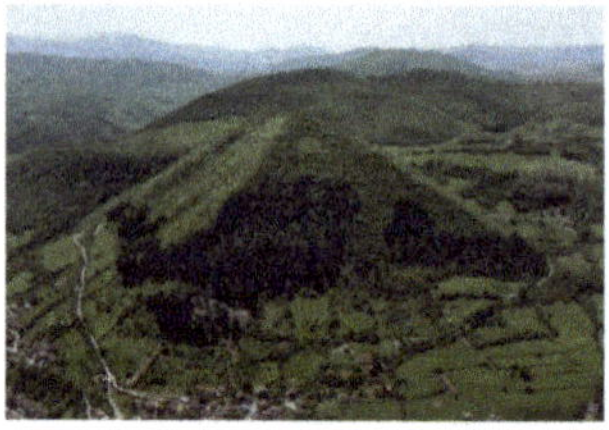

This trituration proving took place on 16 March 2025, from within the Bosnian Pyramid of the Sun in Visoko, Bosnia.

19 provers were involved in the making and proving of this remedy.

There were 17 women and 2 men, and we noted that 19 is the number of spheres that make up the Flower of Life. The provers were mostly students and teachers at the Golden Spiral International School of Homeopathy, joined by 3 friends of the School.

The remedy was triturated to a 12c initially, then 28c at a later date, using the intuitive method of trituration.

The trituration began 48 hours after the Virgo Full Moon and lunar eclipse, so took place as we were emerging out of it. A lunar eclipse brings a sense of completion of a cycle and ushering in a new one.

Key themes astrologically included a Pisces North Node, which according to astrologer Amy Bird encouraged us to find a "greater degree of acceptance, and to forgive ourselves and others for our so-called imperfections. We are only human, and human beings make mistakes sometimes!". Amy went on to describe that the Moon invited us to "embrace the helpful traits of Virgo and develop healthy routines that help us to take care of our mind, body and spirit. Pisces is calling for us to still the monkey mind, open our hearts and connect to the unseen, developing a deeper connection to spirit......This is a great time for meditation, Tai Chi, yoga, prayer and all forms of healing and energy work, especially in the build up to this Moon, as we could be feeling more tender, open and connected to all that is.

Saturn was also sitting right next to the Pisces Sun, opposing the Moon, which Amy explained also called for us to "develop greater discipline and control over ourselves and to set healthy boundaries, but could also make things feel a bit heavy and "real". Pisces is the part of us that can tend to bury our heads in the sand when the going gets tough and may prefer to escape into fantasy land or numb out rather than facing reality. Saturn, however, is the planet of reality and the Lord of Karma, so there is no avoiding things when he is around!"

All of these themes were relevant to this proving and remedy!

About the Bosnian Pyramids

Located in Visoko, Bosnia there are 6 pyramids that have been identified. The largest is the Pyramid of the Sun, and there are also the Pyramid of the Moon, the Pyramid of the Dragon, the Pyramid of Love, the Pyramid of earth and a 6th one that, at the time of writing is as yet unnamed.

The Pyramid of the Sun has remnants of a fortress on the top of it. This is the place where in 1189, Bosnia was created, with the first King being crowned in Visoko. Sarajevo, the nearest city, is known as "the Jerusalem of Europe"; there are 4 religions that co-exist within 400 square metres (Islam, Christian Orthodoxy, Catholicism and

Judaism), so there are strong multi-cultural origins throughout Bosnia.

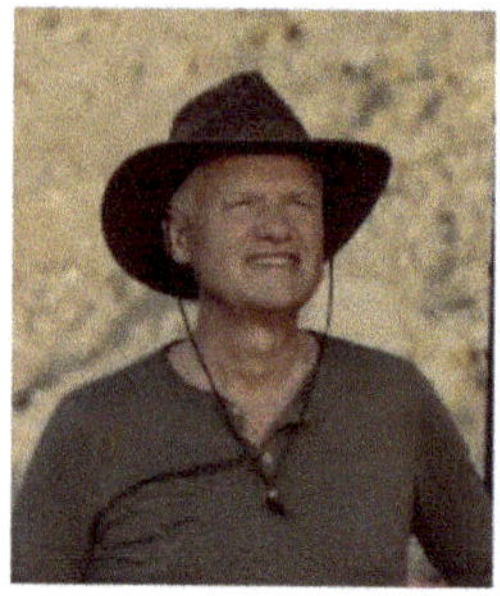

Dr Semir Osmanagich, who has a doctorate in Social Sciences, had been researched and studied archaeological sites including pyramids around the world. He discovered the first pyramid - the Pyramid of the Sun in 2005. Dr Osmaganich himself is Bosnian, but had been living in Houston, Texas in the USA since moving there because of the war in the 1990s.

Due to his interest in archaeological artifacts, he had been invited to Visoko to visit the local museum to see a artifact. He describes how he looked up at the "hill", the highest point in Visoko - Visoko means "high" in Bosnian), and realised that it had four sides, triangular faces and four corners - in other words, that he was looking at a pyramid! Georadar and geothermal imaging helped to confirm that this was indeed a pyramid he had discovered.

Even though the Bosnian Pyramid of the Sun wasn't discovered until 2005, 10 years previously during the war in 1995, local people would describe hearing the resonant sound of bombs landing on the Pyramid, and there being a hollow sound that would then emanate. The incredible strength of the concrete which I will describe later withstood the bombs.

In an interview with *Awakening Times,* Dr Semir Osmaganich describes how "I took a compass and the compass showed me that those four sides perfectly match the cardinal points east, west, north and south. And for 25 years before that, I had been researching pyramids all over the planet. You know how they taught us that pyramids are built only in Egypt and Mexico and that the Egyptian pyramids were built as tombs for Pharaohs. Well, that's wrong. Pyramids have been built all around the planet on all six continents. Probably I'm the person who has visited and investigated most of them; from 250 BC Pyramids in China, Koh Ker pyramids in Cambodia, pyramids in Indonesia, Australia, Sudan, Egypt, Canary Islands, Mauritius, Peru, Bolivia, Mexico, Guatemala, Honduras, El Salvador, Belize, The USA, Spain, Greece and finally Bosnia; most of them are really covered by solid vegetation, just like in Bosnia. I started preliminary research, archaeological digging, geological core drilling and finally, I wrote the book about the discovery of first pyramids in Europe. I established a non-profit foundation for archaeological research. In the last 15 years, it has become the most active archaeological site in the world. Hundreds of volunteers come every year in Bosnia, so far 3500 of them, and they discover with us the oldest concrete blocks from the Bosnian pyramids; the oldest and most extensive underground tunnel network older than 30,000 years, artefacts, energy measurements are showing us that pyramids have benefits to human health. They have very specific frequencies which improve the molecular structure of the water, food, our immunity and they help us to develop our spiritual abilities. This place has become much more than an archaeological site; we have the energy aspect; we have the spiritual aspect; we have the healing aspect.[48]

Dr Semir Osmaganich has remarkably created an area in the war-torn former Yugoslavia to bring together experts and scientists from across the former Yugoslavia - from Croatia, Slovenia, North Macedonia and Serbia, making the Bosnian Pyramids an even more remarkable area of healing and reunification. Serbian tennis star Novak Djokovic has visited several times and paid for a professional tennis court to be built in the grounds in the Pyramid Complex, inviting professional tennis players from around the world to play there. This is also important to note in terms of the proving of the

48 https://awakeningtimes.com/discovering-pyramids-with-dr-semir-osmanagich/

remedy.

The Bosnian Pyramid complex is 30,000 years old with many tunnels underneath them. Scientists and geologists have identified that around 5,000 years ago, the tunnels were filled in. They have no idea how there were filled in, but there is a really interesting monolithic stone with some kind of runic language written on it. Different specialists in runic languages have been consulted to help interpret the message on one particular large stone. The language written on the stone isn't exact to runic languages that are known, but the closest and most similar runic language interpretation of the message on the monolithic stone is that it says:

"The gate is closed. We need to fight and conquer until the gate is open again".

The precise orientation of the Pyramid of the Sun has been measured to be even more accurate than the Great Pyramid of Giza (Cheops) - the deviation from cosmic north with the Bosnian Pyramid of the Sun is only 12 seconds, whereas it is 3 minutes with The Egyptian Cheops pyramid. Whereas the Giza Pyramids are aligned cosmically with Sirius, the Bosnian Pyramids are aligned with the Pleiades.

There is an exact equilateral triangle between the pyramids of the Sun, Moon and Dragon, with each side measuring exactly 2.2m.

The tunnels inside the Pyramids are built to contain a system of lower and higher ceilings, this ensures a constant air flow. Higher ceilings equals lower pressure, and the parts of the tunnels that have lower ceilings mean higher pressure and so they force each other to circulate the air and maintain a healthy air flow.

Inside the tunnels there is a constant vibration of 7.83Hz - the Schumann Resonance of the Earth. In normal everyday life, we may live in cities with a vibration of 30Hz, which is dysregulating for our nervous system. 7.83Hz however is the vibration known as the "heartbeat" of Mother Earth; it is the vibration we experience when we are born, when we meditate, when we are in deep sleep and when in prayer - whatever religion or spiritual practice we might follow, and so being in the vibration of 7.83Hz is regulates the nervous system; much like a distressed baby will be soothed by lying on a mother's chest and hearing and feeling her heartbeat.

Inside the tunnels, there is also a very high level of negative ions. Negative ions combat stress. A city might have 40-200 negative ions per cubic cm (cm3), a forest or the sea might have 1,000-2,000 negative ions per cubic cm (cm3), however inside the Bosnian Pyramids, there can be as many as 18,000 negative ions per cm3 - at least NINE TIMES that of a forest or the seaside!

Many people travel from across the former Yugoslavia, Europe and the World to sit in the tunnels and experience breathing in the negative ions. Whilst no-one working at the Bosnian Pyramids, or indeed Dr Semir Osmaganich can make any claims about the health benefits of visiting the Bosnian Pyramids and sitting in the tunnels, some individuals experience remarkable health benefits.

A 2023 study found that exposure to negative air ions (NAIs) may benefit health by "changing amino acid metabolism, which mainly manifests as increased anti-inflammation and reduced inflammation and antioxidation. Furthermore, exposure to NAIs promotes energy production, affects the expression of c-fos, and regulates 5-HT levels.[49]

49 Xiao S, Wei T, Petersen JD, Zhou J, Lu X. Biological effects of negative air ions on human health and integrated multiomics to identify biomarkers: a literature review. Environ Sci Pollut Res Int. 2023 Jun;30(27):69824-69836. doi: 10.1007/s11356-023-27133-8. Epub 2023 May 12. PMID: 37170052; PMCID: PMC10175061.

5-HT is a precursor to serotonin, the "happiness hormone". c-Fos is "a protein encoded by the c-fos gene, which is an immediate early gene involved in cell proliferation, differentiation, and neuronal activity. It's a proto-oncogene, meaning it can contribute to cancer development if its expression is dysregulated.[50]

There are consistent reports of individuals with high blood pressure or high blood sugar levels experiencing those levels falling significantly and even normalising after drinking water from the Bosnian Pyramids or spending time in the Pyramids.

Sacred Geometry is found throughout all pyramid complexes, including the Bosnian Pyramid complex. This includes the Flower of Life, Golden Spiral, Phi (1.618) and Pi (3.14). This sacred geometry is found throughout the Bosnian Pyramid complex, including a recent discovery that the layout of the different pyramids themselves follows the Golden Spiral, as we also see happens in Giza. Dr Osmaganich describes this in a video he recorded in May 2025.[51]

As I wrote in *Nature's Medicine Code*[52], which was also cited in the Proving Publication of the *Golden Spiral Homeopathic Remedy* that was published in 2021:

"Phi, symbolised by the Greek letter ϕ, has a value of 1.61803399 known as the Golden Number, Golden Ratio or Golden Mean. (or 1.618 for short). It is known as the Golden Number, Golden Ratio or Golden Mean.

Please refer to pages 63-65 for a summary of the Fibonacci

---

50 Velazquez FN, Caputto BL, Boussin FD. c-Fos importance for brain development. Aging (Albany NY). 2015 Dec;7(12):1028-9. doi: 10.18632/aging.100862. PMID: 26684501; PMCID: PMC4712328.
51 https://www.youtube.com/watch?v=b6F0PMjl1i4&t=12s
52 Danica Apolline-Matic *Nature's Medicine Code: Second Edition* (2024) Danica Apolline-Matic (First Edition published in 2018)

Sequence.

During our time with the Pyramids, we were told of the work of Dr Valery Uvarov. He is a Russian scientist who specialises in re-creating pyramid structures and measuring their effects. Whilst I haven't been able to cite the exact research, we were told by the tour guide that he built a pyramid into which he placed some salt and water, which he left for 6 months.

These were then given daily to the most violence prisoners in a prison in Russia where levels of violence had reached 95% for one month. After one month, the levels of violence had reduced to 5%.

Given that pyramid structures contain Phi mathematics (the vibration of love), this would make sense.

So the Bosnian Pyramids, like the Giza Pyramids, have the vibration of love (Phi: 1.618) vibrating through it's complex.

There are several egg-shaped monolithic stones that are made of clay, quartz crystal and sandstone, which will have been smelted together at very high temperatures to form a ceramic - at temperatures of 1000-1500 degrees.

There is a water stream that runs 21m underneath the monoliths. The water produces geopathic waves, so the monolithic stones amplify the vibration of the water that runs The monolithic ceramic stone that we sat and triturated at, K2, is the largest of the monolithic stones, and has extra quartz within it.

The concrete slabs that form the Bosnian Pyramids have a remarkable quality.

The quality of concrete is based on its pressure and water absorption. If concrete absorbs too much water, it freezes as ice in winter then causes the concrete to crack.

Standard concrete can withstand 10-80 mega pascals of pressure and has 3% water absorption.

The best human concrete withstands 110 mega pascals and also has 3% water absorption

The Bosnian Pyramid concrete withstands 155 mega pascals and has only 1% water absorption! Each concrete block is different. The largest block weighs 44.8 tons.

It simply isn't possible that the concrete, and the ceramic monolithic stones, as well as the tunnels are naturally occurring. These have to have been built or created by another civilisation.

Scalar waves, that are 2 million times the speed of light have been measured on each of the Bosnian pyramids. These are known as "Tesla Waves", named after famous Serbian genius Nikola Tesla. Waves usually travel horizontally, however Tesla discovered scalar waves that defy what is understood in physics conventionally; they transmit vertically. This suggests that the Pyramids may have some kind of energy transmitting properties. Dr Semir Osmaganich explains more about them here.[53]

Thank you to all of our amazing provers - students and teachers at the Golden Spiral International School of Homeopathy, and friends of the School: Nicki Miller, Rebecca Dove-Thomas, Ramona Popescu, Rakhee Shah, Jenie Sparkes, Rebecca Westbrook, Natalie Clapham, Michelle Childs, Michelle O'Donnell, Bex White, Gail Shaw, Hayley Hurst, Suzette Knight, Mike Andrews, Peter Angel, Lisa, Bree & Kristina Samoilova.

53 https://www.youtube.com/watch?v=As4flasei08

We would all like to offer our deepest gratitude and appreciation to Dr Semir Osmaganich who brought these incredible Pyramids to the attention of us all, who also made time to personally give us a tour, and for all of his remarkable work, love and dedication, as well to our tour guides, Ajdin Ahmetspahić, Dino and Esmer who so wonderfully took care of us. And an extra special thank you to the wonderful mothers & grandmothers led by beautiful Asma who so lovingly made us all a nourishing feast of Bosnian foods for our lunches whilst we were on our trip - their smiles, and love and generosity were truly appreciated and will be remembered by us all.

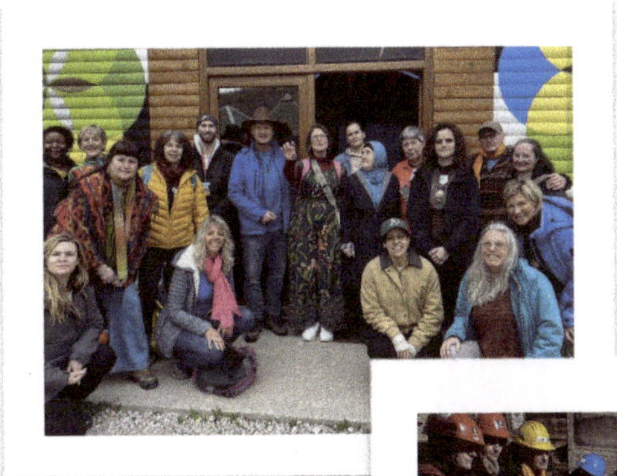

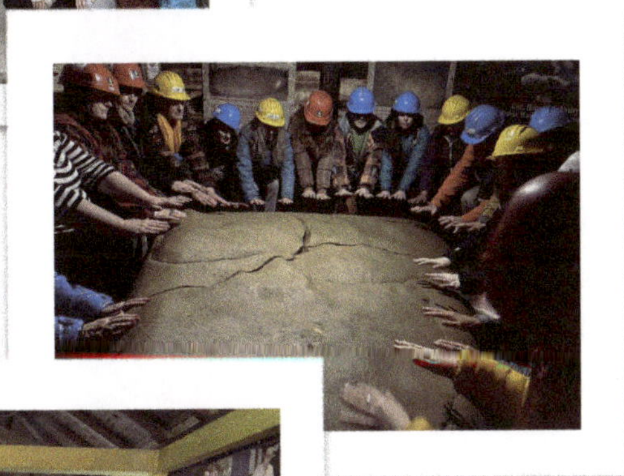

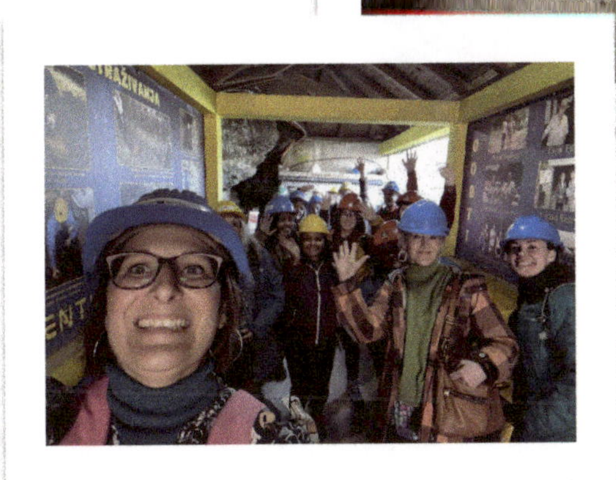

The Bosnian Pyramid of the Sun Homeopathic Remedy™

Key Themes

Peace & Healing - Individual, collective and ancestral
Truth, and shadow to Light
Money
Lost & Found
Clearing out / declutterring / rearranging
Separation
Alignment
Protection
Vision
Telepathy
TIme
Connection
Ease & Flow
We are powerful creators
Spiders
Dragons
Stars
Meditation
Tinnitus
Musculoskeletal (MSK) symptoms
Allergies
Lungs
Heart

Peace & Healing - Individual, collective and ancestral

In keeping with the incredible healing frequencies of the Bosnian Pyramids, this is a remedy that brings tremendous peace and healing - individually and collectively too. It brings a connection to our true self, and who we are. As one prover said:

“When this is used on places where there are places of trauma, it just melts away. It’s like the missing part of our humanity. That connection to the Gods.”

Another prover described feeling a “ total sense of peace throughout the whole process. Felt I could let go of everything, family, work. No thoughts could come in. I could only be present.”. Another said “I have the feeling of not having to be anywhere. Not hurried. Everyone was so present - even the guide. Feeling of being. Not thinking of anything beyond now.” Another said “In the tunnels all thought disappeared and I was just at one with everything, I’d returned to Source."
Some of the individual healing came in the form of realising that it was OK to be ourselves:

“I am dropping a sense of shape. Being loud and raucous and bawdy. I can say what’s on my mind without hurting people. It’s OK to say things, it’s OK to heal.”

One prover was drawn to the crack in the rock (K2). “The crack in things - we discard them.....the crack makes it powerful. Needs to be celebrated, makes it stronger - relates to all of the traumas and brokenness which makes everything so powerful.”

Sometimes the healing felt difficult. One described a “fear of letting go into transformation and change. As speaks it out, everything is relaxing, chest is calming, is coming into peace. It isn’t the big rush I was scared of.”

Some provers connected with the Golden Spiral and the healing energy of it that we find in the Bosnian Pyramids. "We will help our bodies find the light and the road to healing. Spiral of light, lots of golden light."

On a collective level, it was felt that this remedy was the "beginning of a chain reaction bringing peace to the world".

Several provers channelled messages from the beings inside the Bosnian Pyramids, who were also helping us to remember the peace that they are connected with:

"Yes we are the ancient ones but we are of course here now with you and we are so delighted that you have come to this place. Be aware of our bodies, of our lightness, that is here. More than anything it is not words but it is this feeling of group connectedness and of peace, very real deep peace. Peace which you hold in the whole of your bodies and this body becomes a beacon of peace to all that is around you. That is one of the most important things to hold solidly - the frequency of peace. Peace is so filled with love and connection and with being together and as you hold this peace, you hold this frequency, it ripples out to touch and connect all that is around you."

A love of Mama Gaia and a remembering that we are sovereign also came through. It very much felt that the Bosnian Pyramids wished to call us to our sovereignty.

"We have forgotten the beauty of this Earth our Mother and seeing the lushness and green of our planet, and seeing the industrial factories and the smoke billowing out of those factories, and can hear - no! It's time to go back to the beginning and return to our Mother, there has been a thought that we might just leave her and go to other planets and we can travel energetically. It is not for us to escape our planet because we feel she can not sustain life anymore because of our actions, its is for us to heal our division that has led to what has gone on the Earth. We are to return to the old ways, but with a new illumination. Overlay, celebrating the best of the old but with a new vibration. Its is important for us to be. Here, it's in these lands that there is still a reverence for the land and a remembering, to know that we are provided for but not to take out of balance. This remedy will help people know their roots, and live closer to what the Mother gives us. This is a remedy for greed and disharmony and a lack of balance. It's a remedy for unity which is what these pyramids represent. Unity, oneness, love, freedom, sovereignty. I see sovereignty landing through all of those words and anchoring into the Earth. We are sovereign beings and we must remember that this is who we are and what we are."

Ancestral traumas were also also brought to the attention of provers, as they were being healed. One prover said:

"When [we were] talking about [being] sovereign and sovereignty - I could feel chains of slavery falling away, and could feel like a golden being rising up. We are leaving slavery behind."

The power of the Bosnian Pyramids, and this remedy, to bring healing across the collective was so beautifully summarised by the experience of one prover on the plane on the way home.

"On the plane home I sat next to two Muslim guys who'd been back and forth to Bosnia over the last 10 years as part of a multi faith group who deliver aid and support to Bosnian families. They're a group of atheists, Christians, Muslims etc and the work they did was amazing. We spoke for the whole flight and it was amazing, shared what we had been doing and we both said it was too much of a coincidence that we had both been on healing missions and then connected."

This is such a beautiful reflection of Dr Osmaganich's own ethos and work to bring scientists from all over the world, especially from across the whole of the former Yugoslavia - making the Bosnian Pyramids a true expression of the healing power of unconditional love.

The levels of healing were felt very deeply - one prover said she felt her soul was "utterly cleansed".

One prover shared a reading from a book - *Mystery of Light* by James Twyman - which is set in 1994 during the time of war here:

"The main character has a dream, he doesn't know why he has come to Bosnia, but knows he had to come here. He's being chased in a forest, he goes into a building, goes downstairs into ground, sees door with light, when opens door sees a 12 sided room, someone is sitting in there and says "come in" and what this emissary is saying is this. "We gather in many parts of the world where there is conflict and we radiate peace. Groups will come together to do this, we wont need to carry on doing this for much longer. They have been holding this frequency for thousands of years. Now groups are taking this on."

There is an invitation with this remedy to welcome joy and happiness, which healing enables. There were a wonderful series of messages that came through the provers in relation to this:

"I just felt HAPPY"
"We need to make it OK to embrace joy"
"We have lost the art of joy"
"The Universe wants us to be happy"
"JOY at the end of the healing"

Others reported feeling "at home".

"These pillules will be little love bombs to spread through the world"

The day after the remedy was triturated, we all went to Sarajevo, which has seen it's fair share of wars. There is a small bridge over the river where Archduke Franz Ferdinand and his wife were shot and killed in 1914, which was the spark that lit the torch paper that led to the outbreak of WW1.
We all made an emotional journey with the triturated remedy and sprinkled some across the whole area where this occurred.

At the first school weekend following the trip, everyone took part in an exercise that was a remarkable blend of homeopathy for healing with constellations work.

We used some of the triturate of the Bosnian Pyramids remedy that had been triturated to 28c which brings healing across all the layers of consciousness all the way up to the Divine according to the amazing Dr Paul Theriault's teachings.

We placed a giant map of the world on the floor, and invited the students and tutors and our wise grandmothers (our school Board who joined us for the first time) to each take it in turn to honour the countries of their ancestors. In the introduction, I shared how sometimes we don't love where we or our ancestors came from - I gave the examples of how it has been hard at times being a Serb especially because of the wars of the 90s, like how it must be hard being Russian nowadays, or how when I was India I was so sad to see adverts for skin bleach everywhere in South India because the beautiful darker skins of Southern India are not valued.

So each of us in turn held some of the Bosnian Pyramid powder, and said the following:
"Thank you to all of my ancestors who came from ....
Thank you for the codes this ancestral line and these precious lands have given me.

I release any doubts I have ever had about the reasons why I have this lineage and I now and forevermore celebrate all of my ancestral origins and welcome all the codes and blessings from my ancestors".

We then placed some of the powder on the world map on the countries of our origin.

The second part was to name somewhere in the world where we would love to see healing and peace, and to place some of the healing powder on the map there too.

There was a beautiful weaving and connecting between our online and in-person students and tutors - each person in the room would first do this for themselves, and then name one of the online students or tutors who would then express their healing statement and the in-person student or tutor would place the remedy on the map on the online person's behalf, before passing it on to the next person in the room.

Some of the remedy was gifted to the seas, an honouring was given to our star origins, and we also sprinkled healing powder everywhere at the end for all those who live in lands that are not theirs, where they are forced to be, and asked for their freedom and release - especially the children.

So many tears were shed.

At the end of the day, we took the healing powder and offered it to Mama Gaia on UK Mother's Day, as it so happened to be, in the beautiful grounds of the Rudolph Steiner grounds, offering it to all the elements, Earth, Air, Fire (burning some), Water (sprinkling some in the pond), to spirit, light, sound, time and plasma. The 9 elements.

We really came away with a profound and deep healing experience.

Truth, and shadow to Light

This is a remedy that reveals truths and shadow in order to bring it to light. This is part of the deeper healing aspects of this remedy.

One prover said: "I need to share the shadow. [It] feels so unimaginable. So heavy. Sense around the silence - I need to shut my mouth. I feel like I am embodying the shadow - over-responsibility to take it on for others, rather than letting others feel the shadow themselves."

One prover said: "I have had to look at the ways in which I am triggered, and how I deal with those triggers. It's been really uncomfortable, but it's necessary for me to be free."

Hidden family secrets were revealed to some provers.

Another prover described the following. "I have had to take a really long, hard look at my finances. I have had to address why I struggle to understand why I have collected debt. I had a healing after the trip to the [Bosnian] Pyramids, and the healer explained that I had taken on the debt of my ancestors. I remembered that when a parent died, I was left with the debts. I have always blamed myself for not being very good with money, but I discovered I was carrying ancestral debts too, which I then did the work to clear. It's been a very painful time of looking at this in myself, but what I can see is that - finally, almost 25 years after their death - that my life makes sense, and I can see "the light" at the end of the tunnel of dealing with all of this."

The Bosnian Pyramids want us to be powerful - and this can only happen if we clear what is in the way of that. One prover said: "I am being given the words receive your power."

Money

Money was a big theme in this proving in other ways.

One prover described having lots of guilt around money having bought some notebooks just before the trip - and dreading that she had spent too much. She described feeling guilty because she "Needs stuff."

Other provers experienced money flying around and falling:

"Money flew across the garden."
"Money fell out onto ground."
"I got a fraud thing came up on my card, no one took anything. I phoned the fraud department and they said phones weren't working and to call back in an hour."
"My invoice went missing."
"My money situation has descended into a poverty I've not experienced before in my adult life - unsure whether can meet own basic needs and provide for myself."

One prover lost her wallet the night before the trip. "I lost my wallet. Went to bed with no money and no cash. I used cards I hadn't used in a long time, nothing worked. I panicked: "I've no money, I'm going on holiday tomorrow". My husband helped me sort it out.". This prover's panic was about not having back up, worrying about how she would cope.

Another prover was charged extra for a suitcase for being too big. As soon as she got to pyramids, she was contacted by a new client wanting some healing, for that exact amount of money. There was a theme as this example illustrates, of what has been lost being found.

Lost & Found

During the proving, much was lost by so many - relationships, friendships, relatives, money, homes, places of safety and security. There can be an Aurum quality to the loss - the most devastating losses. However there is a "lost and found" element to it too - that which is lost isn't truly lost forever.

This is aligned with how the tunnels had to be sealed and the pyramids were "lost" to the world for 5,000 years until Dr Osmaganich discovered them once more. So there is a finding again, of what wants to be found.

There is a strong syphilitic quality to the remedy, the loss that is experienced can be very destructive and painful to those who might benefit from this remedy.

Twice the actual proving notes were lost (I have never lost proving writings before!) before they were miraculously found.

For one prover, sexual connection with her partner had been lost, and she discovered she was able to experience intimacy with her partner once more.

One prover lost her bag at hotel, but got her bag easily.
Another prover left her passport in an airport toilet, which she wouldn't normally do, and that was easy to get back.

Another prover said: "I have had an influx of new clients and more varied paid work which has been great, much more suited to my current skill set, better paid and drains me less than the other work."

Clearing out / declutterring / rearranging

A big part of the healing, and moving shadow into light involved a good clear out - physically, emotionally, energetically - and with relationships too. For those that have had a Reiki attunement, when an attunement happens, we are told to expect that some relationships may gently fall away, and other soul family members will come in. The emphasis is on the word "gentle".

The clearing out with this remedy is anything but gentle as we found!

Provers said:

"I did a big tidy up before coming out."
"I rearranged my kitchen - I felt good."
"I had people staying so I had to tidy - I was embarrassed for friends to see - feeling the weight of STUFF - this stuff has to be out of my life."
"I also had people staying so had to tidy up."
"It's like I was preparing for something - nesting."
"I'm disgusted with myself that I had let my bathroom get so bad."
"I had a sense of urgency to get everything finished before coming - I did 7 loads of washing."
"I did 6 loads of washing."
"I did LOADS of washing."

One prover's son had gone on a cleaning spree! "He hadn't done the usual clean - it was like he was trying to give himself an energetic clean or energetic reset."

In terms of relationships, a few experienced fallings out with those whom it was no longer a healthy relationship.

"[I had a] huge row with a friend who turned out to be a covert narcissist - who had invaded all aspects of my life, a bit like how [the Serbian Army] surrounded the [Sarajevo] basin and triangulated in that way, it was like an assault."

"[I had a] conflict with a friend from dance who was going to be my second homeopathy patient - entitled, angry, rude to me, brought the personal into the professional, I'd overextended myself and gone out of my way for her and she didn't even appreciate it. This is the end of my over-giving."

Healthier boundaries with family members or friends where there has been enmeshment or a boundary rupture also took place.

One prover reconnected with an old friend where there had been a separation due to a misunderstanding some 20 years previously, and this old friend helped her.

Separation

Part of the theme of loss includes separation from loved ones, in a way that is similar to Berlin Wall.

The tunnels were sealed off to prevent others accessing the Pyramids for 5,000 years. The Bosnian Pyramids have also lived through the War in Yugoslavia, a war which divided and separated families. Many families in the former Yugoslavia were blended culturally. There were families where Bosnians and Serbs had married, others where Bosnians and Croats had married, others still where Croats and Serbs married. Bosnia was at the very centre of Yugoslavia, a country of Slovenians, Macedonians, Croats, Serbs, Montenegrins, Bosnians, with Orthodox Christians, Catholic Christians, Jews and Muslims living together side by side. During the 1990s, the War in Yugoslavia saw a complete rupture of this, and whole families were torn apart and became separated. There were blended families where one member would go to fight for one side, and another member would go and fight for another side - it was a war where it was said that "brothers turned on brothers".

One prover lost her grandmother - her mother's mother, and neither her nor her mother were told for months, and were not allowed to honour her. The other relatives made sure that they took the grandmother's house for themselves.

Another prover had found the need to assert herself in two different friendships in order to protect a project they had worked on. This hadn't been easy for anyone, but the prover felt very strongly that it felt like it happened because there was a protection that was needing to be placed around the project.

One prover described it as follows: "I have noticed a gradual 'quietness' and 'slipping in the background' of a few of what I thought they were my very good friends. I thought they were celebrating my new shift professionally, however, whilst I was being congratulated by so many new friends and amazing people in my life, the old ones chose another position - the background one. Not even a "well done". Nothing....in the end I decided to limit their access to me and my life by taking steps in that direction and blocking them all. Strangely enough, I feel liberated." The same prover also blocked an ex who had been trying to re-establish contact in a way that didn't respect her boundaries.

This takes us back to the Key Theme of "Lost and Found" - that was in lost is what is no longer congruent or aligned, however what is found is freedom, liberation, safety, clarity, self-respect and direction.

Alignment

Underpinning these themes are 2 aspects - alignment and protection.

Alignment, which is the major key theme of the Golden Spiral, emerged again and again as a key theme with this remedy too.

Whereas the Golden Spiral brings a gentle alignment, the Bosnian Pyramid remedy has a much stronger aspect to it how it brings alignment, and so isn't quite so easy or comfortable for everyone.

One prover said:

"Clarity of self has happened and I feel myself coming deeply into alignment with my mission in life and all that I can be. A lot more feels possible and I am very happy with the transformation taking place in myself and my life. Beautiful!"

Protection

Ultimately, provers that experienced a destructive end to certain relationships or situations felt that this had happened because they were being brought an additional level of protection.

The tunnels had been filled 5,000 years ago and it was felt that "there is this desire to speak about the tunnels and it feels like they [filled the tunnels] because we weren't ready, they wanted to protect the vibrations and the integrity of the vibration. It feels like someone would have come and damaged and blown up the pyramids so they filled the tunnels in so no one could destroy the tunnels."

One prover was shown that "during the bombing in the 1990s there was an energetic shield that came to protect the pyramids, the beings that protect the pyramids put in this extra layer. These are very protected their is a real commitment to keep them safe, they would rather it be close than have.

As one prover said: "People, places and things not in alignment are being ripped from me somewhat viciously, kinda painfully really, feels like war."

We are reminded of how the Pyramids just weren't damaged by the wars of the 1990s, even though local residents knew when the Pyramid had been hit because they could hear a "hollow" sound created when a bomb landed.

It feels like this remedy literally stops the destruction of what needs protecting, but is fierce in how it protects.

Vision

This is a remedy that enhances vision and intuition - "it will help inner and outer vision - it will help to see and known with clarity what is to be seen and known
It is different for each one of you. You don't have to strive for that knowing."

"I can SEE things in the field, sometimes comes with words, visions or feelings."

"Physical body is here, but energetic body is somewhere else."

Telepathy

Several provers experienced telepathy.
"When someone says something, I can instantly feel what they are saying and see what they say."

"Extra sensory perception has been at its peak since the trip, I just KNOW things now, like very certain."

Time

Time was a really big theme with this remedy. As one prover described:

"Time seem to be elongated during the trip. I remember when we were in the tunnels triturating I think we were in the for over 2 hours, maybe close to 3 hours, but to me it only felt like about 30mins. The actual trip wasn't even a whole week, but to me it felt like we were there in Bosnia for at least 2 weeks.

To add to that, I feel like something happened with time over this past weekend. I went to an event on Friday evening, it honestly feels like that was weeks ago. Even when we arrived at school on Saturday morning, it didn't feel like the event was only the night before. So much so that I feel like I'm starting to forget it already as if it was weeks or months ago.

Also, it doesn't feel like we were at school this weekend. I know consciously that we were and that I saw everyone yesterday, but it feels like that was weeks ago."

Another said: "Time stretched, it felt like we were there a week and was only 4 days."

Connection

We all felt an immense sense of connection throughout this trip - to each other, to the Pyramids, to our guides, and also to something much bigger.

The number 22 was a big theme, many of us kept seeing 22 - in fact we travelled from Gate 22!

We got cars from Car Genie and we were driving Skoda Karma cars.

Several provers (many!) felt chatty to everyone else like best friends. One said:
"There is a sense of ease and connection, I am never like that normally."

Another said: "I am usually a shy person, but I was very chatty, it was much easier to speak with people that I didn't know (including strangers). I was able to speak in large groups that I found very difficult previously. I didn't hold back, said what I wanted to say, sharing was easy."

There was a lot of laughter - belly laughs even.

People saw a deepening of existing connections, some of which is linked to the "Lost and Found" theme. As one prover said: "Friendships have got better and deeper, I am relying on people more, I am opening up to people more."

One said: "As I stepped into the tunnels MY DAD SENT ME A MESSAGE SAYING HAVE A GOOD DAY, LOVE YOU! And he has been more active on text. Very very random and cosmic."

Ease & Flow

Whilst there is a deep clearing and re-aligning aspect to this remedy, some of which is very uncomfortable, the journey is to get to a place of ease and flow.

One prover had technical challenges with checking in online, and couldn't get insurance working. Many others reported how "everything was smooth and in flow" - especially in terms of the journey.

"All obstacles taken out of my hands and dealt with."

We are powerful creators

We were reminded that we are powerful creators.

In going through the airports, two refused to go through the scanners. One, who believe she would go through easily, did. Another who expected it to be difficult, experienced it being difficult.

Spiders

We all saw so many spiders! In fact there was a spider that came down from the tunnel ceiling, right in front of us, whilst we were triturating! There is definitely a spider theme to this remedy, but not in the way of spider remedies homoeopathically, but in more esoteric ways.

Spiders weave their webs by launching themselves into the aether and catching on the energy lines that make up the energy field we find ourselves in. It felt like our seeing spiders connected with this reminder of our ability to weave energy.

Also spiders can represent luck and it felt that this was the message of the spiders we were seeing.

Dragons

Many provers felt a dragon energy throughout the trip, and in the tunnels. One prover described seeing a "huge lizard like creature, has gone more dragon as I have started speaking. Feels very wise. Curious. I feel like it's deep in the earth. It's female."

One prover saw a dragon in a cave, and wanted to giggle and smiled. Another saw a red dragon, and another saw a pile of golden dragon eggs.

Stars

The Bosnian Pyramids have a huge connection to the stars and to the Cosmos.

During the proving, some felt a connection to Atlantis. As one prover said: "Atlantis in its heyday, when everything was in balance, the beautiful technologies, love, peace."

Several provers described becoming really long, with elongated faces, and with the spine being pulled up into alignment.

Of all of the physical symptoms, by far the most reported were symptoms connected with the musculoskeletal system - and one aspect of this was the spine being pulled into alignment.

The spine - and all of the bones - are crystalline in nature, and actually look like a tuning fork when we look at it, with the skull being the "handle" or top of the fork. The crystalline bones are crucial for receiving information from the cosmos. When the spine is not in alignment, we can't receive all that we need to, and it felt very much that we were being adjusted and pulled into alignment - and this can help us to receive more from the cosmos.

Some of us saw other provers looking like a star version of themselves.

Other saw star beings around us. Some of what was shared includes:

"They are being really playful and light on their feet. Inquisitive."
"It looks full of joy. It's gorgeous gorgeous gorgeous light."
"I am feeling a lot of joy because there is a star being here. I can really see them. They are really long. Not tall, just long."
"They need the joy to connect. The happier we are, the easier it is to connect"

Some felt that we were being downloaded codes. Others experienced a connection between the Pyramids and the Stars. "I feel like I can travel into the underground where all the creatures are, and back to the stars", one prover shared.

One of the provers described what Dr Semir Osmaganich talks about in terms of Tesla's scalar waves that travel vertically up and out of the Pyramids, defying the laws of physics as we know them - that the Pyramids were a means of communicating with the stars.

"Meditation in afternoon: Went deep in quickly, could see pyramid as it was before growth on it. Purpose was to communicate with stars and ETs. Shown a HUGE pyramid - could see the top of it covered in snow, was told it was in the Himalayas - Nepal/Tibet."

Another, whilst in meditation saw a pyramid with a golden spiral coming down the pyramid.

"This is a remedy that goes through time and space, connects us with all other civilisations in all time and space. We can take this remedy when we would like to ask questions. Seek and ye shall find."

One prover felt like her skin boundary was merging with a oneness, she felt like she didn't have an edge or a contour, which can be very star-like.

Sound

We now live in a time when we all understand the importance of sound as an expression of energetic frequencies - and the ability of harmonious sounds to bring healing and activations.

One prover experienced the sound vibrations of the whales and dolphins whilst in the tunnels. It is said by some who follow starseed influencers that dolphins and whales are connected to the stars, and have come from and express frequencies of the stars on Earth.

Another prover thought about sound chambers in sacred places all over the world. "There is a way in which sound travels through this place" was shared.

Another observed how the DNA - the spiral of the DNA - changed with the sound sitting in the Pyramids, even though we couldn't audibly hear a sound.

Meditation

It was very much felt that this would be a good remedy to take before meditating, due to the high frequencies, and connections with sacred geometry and the stars that the Pyramids connect us with.

Physical Key Themes

Tinnitus

Two provers found their tinnitus disappeared. One had had tinnitus for 8 years and sometimes hadn't been able to sleep because of how loud it had been, and it was in both ears. She realised during meditation in tunnels, that she wasn't able to hear it. "It was so quiet and peaceful", she said.

Back, Spine & Musculoskeletal (MSK) Symptoms

Almost every imaginable symptoms relating to the MSK system presented itself. There were consistent reports of the spine being pulled into alignment, and of pains leaving the body.

One prover said: "I felt an involuntary lift from my chest, and my whole spine straighten, from here I am being pulled up - it's like having an adjustment. I came back down and the spine is correcting itself. Something is really releasing, through my spine and neck. Something is wanting to release. Lots of crying as a result."

Allergies

This is a remedy to consider for allergies, even if as a support remedy alongside others.

Lungs

This is a remedy that can be considered for those with asthma, even

if as a support remedy alongside others, including Flower of Life.
Heart

This is a remedy that can be considered for regulating blood pressure, and how oxygen is carried within the blood (anaemia).

Mental & Emotional Symptoms

Lack of self-love
Self-doubt
Shadow work
Reluctance for transformational work
Ungrounded
Not present
Hurried - too much to do
Fear of letting go into transformation and change
Difficulties letting go into intimacy with partner
Cringing when being sexually touched - even if by a loving partner
Loss of property (Aurum)
Fear of having no money
Panicky
Overwhelmed
Fearful about what might lose, or has lost
Difficulties speaking in groups of people
Fear around speaking, feeling silent
Shyness
Huge grief
Wailing for the Earth
Sorrow and deep lament for what has gone on with the Earth (Thymus Gland)
Feeling the trauma in the Earth
Feeling rage at what has been done to our beautiful planet
Syphilitic levels of loss and destruction
Fear of dying

Fear of what might happen to children, when leaving them
Anticipatory anxiety (Arg nit)
Sloppiness and clumsiness - things falling out
Feeling exceptionally tall / long
Claustrophobia
Feeling intoxicated
Feeling soft like Mr Soft
Imprisonment (physically, mentally, emotionally or spiritually) (Goldfish)
Anger (Ignatia)
Feeling stuck
Conflict in family - including siblings, may be very destructive
Extreme tiredness
No energy
Fed up
Demotivated
Getting cross over little things
Impatient
Concentration - lack of
Isolated
Wanting freedom
Hard to find joy
Wanting to be with tribe
Burdened
Carrying weight
Unsettled
Destabilised
Lethargic
Addictions

"Give remedy during detox will help integrate the new feelings so they can keep going and not be in fear, it softens everything ANY FORM OF TRANSFORMATION THEY ARE TRYING TO MAKE, REHABILITATION they can keep going on that journey and see it through."

Physical Particulars

Head

Head feels really heavy

Eyes

Poor vision - can see more clearly
Lack of vision in right eye
Lachrymation
Allergic responses

Ears

Tinnitus
Heard a high pitched sound towards the end
Pain in left ear
Left ear blocked
Pressure in right ear

Nose

Coryza
Coryza, clear, left nostril
+++ Sneezing
Allergic responses
Sinus infection
Sinus pain or blockage
Hayfever symptoms

Mouth & Teeth

+++ dry mouth (thirst)
Sensitive teeth
Trembling jaw
Twitching in lip - right side

Throat

A silencing
Throat has been constricted
Dust in throat
Dry throat
Lump in throat as if food is stuck

Cough

Cough from vinegar
Difficulty clearing using cough - something not releasing
Coughing due to something not being expressed
Cough with copious sputum (clear, bright yellow or green)
Cough with copious amounts of blood caused by the trauma to the back of the throat

Lungs & Breathing

Difficulties breathing
Shallow breathing
Shallow breathing due to anaemia
Shuddering in breathing as though been crying loads
Chest infection
Green, white or mustard bright yellow sputum

Heart & Blood

Anaemia
Haemorrhage
Blockages
Atherosclerosis
Feeling pulse within body
Flutter
Palpitations

Kidneys, Bladder, Urination

Urine - orange
Acute or chronic cystitis
Pain in kidneys (with flu-like symptoms)

Digestion

+++++ gas
Poor digestion
Urgency - no 2
Insatiable hunger
Feeling unsatisfied after food
Nausea
Burping
Belching
Parasites / parasite cleansing
Constipation

Female

Difficulties with intimacy with partner
Can recoil from sexual touch of loving partner
Pain in lower womb
Pain in area where c-section scar location
Pain in left ovary

Back & Limbs

Swollen ankles
Swollen body
Swollen knees, full of fluid
Can hear fluid moving/cracking in knee
Cracking joints
Misalignment structurally
Misaligned spine
Needing spinal corrections, osteopathy
Buzzing in fingers
Tips of fingers all cold
Buzzing in legs
Pain left knee
Pain anywhere in body
L leg feels cold above the knee.
Pain on RHS of body, down hip
Pins and needles in the hands
Pain in knees, feet and heels
Achilles tendon
Body jerking, twitching, involuntary movements
Uncontrollable body movements
Sharp pain, right ankle
Strong pain in right shoulder
Sciatica - left side
Shivers in bottom of back
Lack of flexibility
Carpal tunnel
Muscle loss

Physical Generals

Swollen body
Fluid retention in whole body
Bloating in hands and feet and whole body
Any pain wherever it is in the body

Body Temperature

Extremes of temperature - either very hot or very cold
Hot hands
Vibration through hands

Dreams

Several provers had bad dreams of disasters or some kind of destruction:

"I was waving my arms around, I was shouting "we are on fire! We are on fire!" I could see smoke. didn't realise where I was, then realised I was in the hotel. My heart was hammering, and it took ages to calm my heart down."

"I dreamt of someone I know. In the dream he had terminal cancer. I was trying to attend an event to celebrate him before he died, but I wasn't allowed to attend it by others. I wasn't welcome, or recognised. There would be no reason in the real world for my being excluded were such a situation to arise."

"I dreamt about robbers".

"I am in my grandparents house (Mum's side) - massive rave. All uni friends gathering. All Uni friends sat in sofas randomly eating food. Best friend crushed between sideboard and chair. I went outside. Group of boys, one was really aggressive and was trying to hit and hurt me. I was trying to persuade him to do something else. Went on for about an hour. Eventually I said "look, I'm too old for this. My nervous system can't handle it." And then he went away. Then a young boy chased me, trying to attack and hurt me."

"It was really windy. Shed in garden blew away. Man tried to hold on a canoe. Moved onto being in a cafe with dog. Someone was talking and saying really horrible things about ex-partner. Ex-partner's current partner came out and was looking at me really horribly. Things you think but would never say."

One prover had a dream about truths being revealed. "I was walking around in my swimming costume, belly hanging down to knees, boobs hanging down. Felt like was being told a truth without any negativity behind it. Didn't feel derogatory. Felt refreshing."

Food & Drink

++++ thirsty
Dry mouth (thirst)

Energy

Low energy
Fatigue
Exhaustion

Other

Mould toxicity, mould allergies
++++ yawning
Yawning with whole body
Pain in left lymph - under armpit
Remedy for premature babies to come into plane when reluctant to

incarnate

"This remedy will enhance any other treatment. It's a facilitator."

Modalities

Better rocking
Better swaying

Esoteric

"Purity. So much purity in the room. Energy feels really pure and high."
"Atlantis in its heyday, when everything was in balance, the beautiful technologies, love, peace."
"We are in our New Earth. That Magic Forest, a complete surprise, all the flowers were so beautiful, the veils were so thin."
"Shedding of layers run the yawning. This remedy brings us back to our core."
"For relationships where twin soul is a runner."
"A sense of incredible sense of Light coming through. Illumination."
"We are connected from the belly of the earth, really grounding."
"I am seeing the umbilicus - the energy moving up like an umbilicus"

There is lots of grounding with this remedy.
Opening up of spiritual energy
Vortex of energy felt during proving
Vision of 2 pyramids, with a lot of spirals and a lot of golden light.
Feels lots of expansion, things getting clear. Lots of energy

We travelled from Gate 22.
We hired cars from Car Genie

We are driving Skoda Karma cars
Saw a rainbow just before landing (double rainbow)

Many of us heard songs including:

It's a wonderful life
Scorpio "Take me to the rhythm"
Inner City: Pennies from Heaven ("brothers, sisters.....we need some love")

Chakras

Crown

Crown chakra opening, opening mind
Feels like head opening like a flower. Feels solid. Inflow and outflow - the inflow is making the person feel very grounded

Third Eye

Intense pressure on third eye as though someone pressing
Another prover felt sensation on third eye
Another felt like the third eye was more open than it was moment ago, crystals energy really nice, joyful feeling, middle of head

Throat

The Bosnian Pyramids remedy gives us the energy to speak our truth honouring our boundaries, sometimes with strength and with a protective quality to it, which can be powerful but can create discomfort where there is an imbalance.

The remedy opens the throat chakra so that there is a full expression of anything unexpressed or suppressed. This can include speaking more easily in ways that bring closer and deeper friendships and relationships, and make general communication and chatting easier (Blackbird).

Heart

Lots of energy around the heart chakra, clearing and healing.
Joy coming in

Solar plexus

Heavy feeling in solar plexus, like a ball.

Sacral

This chakra is all about relationships with others. Burning in this chakra. Creativity comes into this chakra too. This remedy opens us up to our creativity

Root

It is a grounding remedy, like Oak, Thuja, Petrified Sequoia & T-Rex.

Remedy Affinities

Argentum nitricum (anticipatory anxiety)
Aurum (loss of property)
Ayahuasca (karmic clearing)
Berlin Wall (war trauma, separation)
Blackbird (Speaking up, with love)
Carcinosin (drawing boundaries)
Chalice Well Water (deep grief)
Flower of Life (lungs, breathing, sacred geometry)
Golden Spiral (sacred geometry, alignment, clearing war trauma,

peace and calm)
Ignatia (anger, grief)
Lotus (stillness, calm, peace)
Oak (grounding, aligning, balancing, unifying)
Petrified Sequoia (ancestral trauma, curses)
Psorinum (fear of loss of property, stability)
Thuja (revealing, uncovering, grounding, detoxification)
Thymus Gland (state of the world)

Case Studies

1) A patient came to me with the request to **open up more to spirituality** and to experience a sense of **clearing**. She mentioned that certain unclear and confusing situations were unfolding in her life. We set an intention for clarity and inner purification.

What followed was both powerful and unexpected: the remedy **brought her back to her fear**—a fear that had remained after a serious illness.

She had been diagnosed with cancer in the past and had gone through healing. However, after taking the remedy, old symptoms reappeared in a way that mirrored her original healing process back in 2019.

"My tongue became so swollen that I bit it involuntarily. I felt pain in my spine and chest..."

These returning symptoms had a purpose: they pointed her back to the **root of her fear** and allowed it to rise to the surface.

As she described, energy naturally flows where attention is directed. This fear had been **unconscious**—she wasn't actively thinking about it. But with the acceptance of the remedy, **it emerged from deep within**.

She realised that this fear must be **faced and healed**, even though it's a journey that takes time.

"I know this isn't something that will be resolved in just one day. But the fact that it came up so clearly showed me it's the key issue I need to work with."

She shared that even before the official diagnosis, she had **self-diagnosed**, carrying a deep **fear of cancer** for years.

"I felt something was wrong as early as 2016. The diagnosis came in 2019."

Now, something within her has shifted. A new internal message has arisen:

"It's time to stop merely surviving and start living." (KS)

2) **Another client, who has been living with ADHD, reported a deeply moving experience after taking the Bosnian Pyramid remedy. She shared the following:**

"At first, when I started the remedy, I felt very emotionally sensitive—even a bit anxious. I was feeling everything very deeply, and many memories started coming back. I began to see some things with fresh eyes."

Her emotional sensitivity initially brought up intensity, but it also allowed for a richer appreciation of life:

"I felt even more joy from life's little pleasures—like nature, the sound of birds, and time spent with the people I love."

Although the emotional process was not always easy, it eventually brought her to a state of balance:

"Some of the effects I experienced while taking the remedy felt intense or difficult emotionally, but now I have a great sense of peace."

The remedy also affected her physically:

"At the start, my energy levels dropped, and I felt fatigued. But after a while, my body and mind felt activated in a new way."

Looking back, she recognises a deep release:

"I think this remedy helped me release some old energy that was stuck—and now, I feel freer and lighter."

This **case** illustrates how energy-based remedies can work on **multiple levels**—emotional, physical, and spiritual to support transformation, especially in people navigating neurodivergent conditions like **ADHD. (KS)**

The Pleiades

18 August 2025
Uluru
Northern Territory
Australia

and 21 December 2025

There were 8 provers in Australia, all were women. A further proving took place on 21 December 2025.

The Pleiades

I have been fascinated with the Pleiades for many, many years. We have been taught that there are, in essence, two theories of the existence of humans - that we came from Adam & Eve, or evolved from monkeys. We haven't been taught the third possibility - and I believe truth - that we came from the stars.

The evidence of this is clear - from the long, elongated skulls and almond-shaped eyes of the Hathors - the first Ancient Egyptians, to crop circles, and all sorts of extraterrestrial phenomena.

The Pleiades is star system that I hear many people describe as a place that feels is home - particularly for those that identify as *starseeds* - those that just *know* lifetimes have been lived in other star systems; on other planets. Starseeds are those who recognise a wisdom and intelligence from the stars.

The Pleiades is commonly known as "The Seven Sisters" - because of the seven brightest stars that can be seen with the naked eye in the night sky. However there are over 200 stars in the Pleiades cluster.

It is said that the Lemurians - a pre-Atlantean civilisation - came to Earth from the Pleiades, bringing with them the Pleiadian gifts of being great healers & teachers. Being deeply intuitive and compassionate, Pleiadian starseeds can absorb the energies of others, and so learning self-care and healthy boundaries can be really helpful.

The Pleiades is said to be a place of learning healing approaches, and also how to transcend limitations, to transmute and transform them, and in so doing connect to a truly higher dimension conscious way of living.

When I began this journey that started with with the Golden Spiral Homeopathic Remedy, I didn't know then that we were being taken on a journey that would lead us to the Pleiades.

It was an intuition that we were to go and make a homeopathic remedy at the Bosnian Pyramids. There, we were blessed to meet Dr Semir Osmaganich, who discovered the Bosnian Pyramids. The Golden Spiral is woven into the entire Bosnian Pyramid complex in the most remarkable ways. We learned when we were there that the Bosnian Pyramids are aligned with the Pleiades star system. When I shared with him my work on the Bosnian Pyramid of the Sun Homeopathic Remedy with Dr Osmaganich, he then informed me that he had just published his remarkable paper proving, for the first time, that the Pleiades star system also aligns with the Golden Spiral.[54]

We had already planned and set the dates to travel to Uluru and the Northern Territory and to make a remedy there. I didn't know what our journey would be, or what remedies we would be making until a week before we were departing, when Dr Osmagaich had emailed

---

54 Osmanagich, S. (2025). Golden Geometry Revealed: The Fibonacci Link Between the Pleiades and the Bosnian Pyramids. Int J Aerosp Sci Technol Engg, 1(1), 01-22.

me the link to his newly published paper, and I shared this with the group travelling, and my dear friend and colleague Nicki Miller messaged and said "is that the remedy we are making?". And then two or three days before departing, I understood that we were also to triturate the sacred geometry remedies.

What is amazing to me is - having travelled to Indigenous lands in Australia, and heard about the Dreaming stories of the Pleiades as told by the Indigenous peoples, is that this is the perfect remedy to bring us full circle with the journey with the Sacred Geometry remedies.

The Original People of Australia all have their own variations of the story of the Pleiades depending on which people are telling the story, in which language, and from which part of Australia. There are variations in the names and details, and we only know a brief summary as these stories are sacred to the Indigenous people; the details of which are protected, usually by senior women. There is however a general summary and similarity in the stories of the Pleiades that we can share.

In Aṉangu Pitjantjatjara Yankunytjatjara land, the lands to which we had travelled, the Seven Sisters are known as Kungkarangkalpa, and their pursuer Wati Nyiru. In accounts, the Kungkarangkalpa flee south from Irawa Bore, a site near Watarrka (King's Canyon), which we were blessed to visit.[55]

Travelling south from the Northern Territory, the Seven Sisters encounter a writhing multicoloured snake-like object. Quickly, the older sister kicks it away, revealing it as the long penis of Wati Nyiru, which he had sent for them in lust. Wati Nyiru continues to pursue them, using an ability to shapeshift to tempt the women as a shady tree and bush food, although he fails to trick the older sister. At

55 Neale, Margo, ed. (2017). *Songlines: Tracking the Seven Sisters*. National Museum of Australia Press

times, his lust becomes a multi-coloured rainbow across the sky, from where he spies. The women interacted with him, at times cheekily, and other times with fear. Several times he uses magic to make them tired. At the cave Walinynga (Cave Hill), Wati Nyiru catches up to them, and they barely escape as his penis, in excited lust, breaks through a wall. Frustrated, Wati Nyiru sings magic, causing the older sister to bleed and fall sick. The sisters become separated for a time as Wati Nyiru catches and attacks her, leaving her bleeding to death. The sisters lift her into the sky and follow her, becoming the star cluster Pleiades. Wati Nyiru continues his chase, becoming the constellation Orion.[56]

I am fascinated by how the Pyramids of Giza align with Orion, and Pyramids of Bosnia align with the Pleiades.

I am also fascinated by the key themes; how the sisters are chased and how they become separated. To me, I see the story of the patriarchy; the divide and conquer approach we see used. In time, there is a reunification of the sisters.

One final aspect of these connections is that the Bosnian Pyramids are located in the home of my ancestors - in the former Yugoslavia.

A country that was once made up of seven provinces, that was manipulated by external influences into war, and became separated.

There are many, many people from the former Yugoslavia who are doing wonderful work to bring healing and peace and to reunite the peoples. My ancestry is Serbian, Montenegrin (and I think a little Bosnian too), but I feel I am with brothers and sisters when I am with Slovenes, Croats, Herzegovians and Macedonians. Dr Semir

56 James, Diana; Williamson, Inawinytji (2017). "So everyone can see: Kungkarangkalpa *inma* in Canberra". In Neale, Margo (ed.). *Songlines: Tracking the Seven Sisters*. National Museum of Australia Press

Osmaginch is one of my personal heroes, because he has intentionally welcomed scientists and people from across the former Yugoslavia to work together to uncover the mysteries of the Bosnian Pyramids; amplifying the healing capacity of the pyramids for the benefit of all of the people of the whole region - and extending into the world.

I believe the story of the Pleiades is the story of the former Yugoslavia - held within the Golden Spiral which is here to realign and bring healing.

It's not just a story told in these areas. This ultimately is the story that we see around the world where manipulations are used to divide peoples and lands.

My sincerest hope and wish as I share this final remedy in the series is that this remedy, and all of these remedies are able to play their part in bringing healing to our beautiful world.

Pleiades Homeopathic Remedy™

Key Themes

Separation from community & kin
Exclusion / inclusion
Affected by external energies
Division to Re-unification
Abuse
Healing
Re-unification
Cosmic knowledge of healing

Separation from community & kin

During this proving, and the journey with this remedy, separation from community was a theme that was present - in fact, the entire story as told by the Original People was very much present in the field.

Exclusion / inclusion

Exclusion / inclusion are a core part of the telling of the story of the Seven Sisters, and we see this replicated.

Affected by external energies

This is particularly helping for those who have been affected by external energies that aren't connecting with the pure unconditional love of Source - energies of manipulation, coercion, gaslighting.

Division to Re-unification

Division Is also fundamental to the energy of the Pleiades - and from this, a journey back to Re-unification with those whose soul journeys are meant for togetherness and unity. This may not apply to every division or separation. I am reminded of the saying:

I am reminded of these wise words by Brian A. "Drew" Chalker

People always come into your life for a reason, a season and a lifetime. When you figure out which it is, you know exactly what to do. When someone is in your life for a REASON, it is usually to meet a need you have expressed outwardly or inwardly. They have come to assist you through a difficulty, or to provide you with guidance and support, to aid you physically, emotionally, or even spiritually. They may seem like a godsend to you, and they are. They are there for a reason you need them to be. Then, without any wrong doing on your part or at an inconvenient time, this person will say or do something to bring the relationship to an end. Sometimes they die, Sometimes they just walk away. Sometimes they act up or out and force you to take a stand. What we must realize is that our need has been met, our desire fulfilled; their work is done. The prayer you sent up has been answered and it is now time to move on.When people come into your life for a SEASON, it is because your turn has come to share, grow, or learn. They may bring you an experience of peace or make you laugh. They may teach you something you have never done. They usually give you an unbelievable amount of joy. Believe it! It is real! But, only for a season. And like Spring turns to Summer and Summer to Fall, the season eventually ends.LIFETIME, relationships teach you a lifetime of lessons; those things you must build upon in order to have a solid emotional foundation. Your job is to accept the lesson, love the person/people (anyway);, and put what you have learned to use in all other relationships and areas in your life. It is said that love is blind but friendship is clairvoyant. Thank you for being part of my life.....

This is a remedy for those that have been divided for whom the story arc of their relationship is for togetherness in the end.

Abuse

Where the remedy Columba (pidgeon) is the bird kingdom equivalent of Staphysagria in the plant kingdom, the Pleiades is the energetic blueprint equivalent.

This is a remedy to welcome healing, and the return of support from those around a person for anyone who has experienced abuse, be it sexual, physical, emotional or spiritual.

Healing

There is deep healing in this remedy.

Cosmic knowledge of Healing

The Pleiades is said to be a place of great knowledge about energy and healing.

Mental & Emotional Symptoms

Feeling like the Earth is not home
Yearning for home
Homesickness
Difficulties understanding life on Earth
Enjoys looking at stars
Find life on Earth hard
Fascinated by aliens
Fascinated by the cosmos
May feel they are a starseed
Feeling different to other people
Feeling misunderstood
Feeling misunderstood
Natural healing abilities
Abuse - mental, physical, emotional, spiritual
Separation from community
Excluded from communities / family
Sensitive to other people's energies
Sensitive to unkind behaviours
Logical thinking
Ungrounded

Physical Particulars

Head

Tingling on top of head
Light feeling in head

Eyes

Sensation of eyes feeling big
Photophobia

Ears

Tinnitus
Pressure in left ear

Nose

Sensitive sense of smell - especially to toxic smells

Throat

Ned to clear throat regularly

Lungs & Breathing

Better open cool air

Back & Limbs

Growing pains
Pains in bones in limbs
Misalignment with skeleton

Atlas bone misaligned
Sensation of limbs feeling long

Physical Generals

Body Temperature

Chilly

Sleep

Waking 3-4am, cannot easily go back to sleep

Dreams

Dreams of the stars
Travelling through the cosmos
Speaking with beings from the stars

Food & Drink

Thirsty

Energy

Generally good energy
When tired needs to rest (Phos)

Modalities

Better cool air
Better evening

Clinical

Autism

Remedy Affinities

Bosnian Pyramid of the Sun
Dodecahedron
Golden Spiral
Hydrogenium
Metatron's Cube
Phosphorus

Provings & The Fabric of The Universe

A realisation about provings unfolded in the journey following the making of these remedies.

Making a new remedy, particularly triturating it in a pestle and mortar, or proving a remedy, opens us up new knowledge, new insights, it transforms what is in physical material form (if not an imponderable) and we experience it's expansion into its energetic counterpart.

It is an amazing medicine we are working with. To do this work, we are alchemists, altering the very nature of a substance, or working with an energetically altered substance in order to prove it.

This is a bit like being a scientist in a laboratory and blowing things up to see what an experiment or a new substance can do. I have discovered the hard way that, as much as a gift it is to be truly in service to homeopathy and our world to do this work, it also can be a challenge. Often there is joy and wonder at the revelations of what a remedy can do. Sometimes however, great sacrifices are made in order to learn about a remedy for the benefit of others, and pain and suffering can be part of the trituration and proving process.

We are exploring the different energetic levels of a substance, and in the process of discovering what it can help with, we are blowing holes in the fabric of reality in order to understand them.

It's a bit like an analogy I will share from some of my favourite books - *His Dark Materials* by Philip Pullman. The books tell of a remarkable parallel reality - and how in the second book in the trilogy *The Subtle Knife* the two main characters Lyra from this parallel reality, and Will from ours, travel together between worlds.

Will, the bearer of the Subtle Knife, can cut through the fabric of the Universe, and can create an opening between worlds. What it also does is that these openings allow energies to also travel between worlds, which isn't always helpful Will is taught how how to close the openings that are made by the Subtle Knife, to keep them safe.

I would suggest that we have, since Dr Hahnemann's day, been blowing up the fabric of reality; of the Universe. We have been in a soup of provings since Dr Hahnemann's time. How many of the challenges that we face can be explained by us being in a proving? We don't even have to be consciously part of the proving, but because we are in a collective consciousness of a profession in which there are constant provings going on. As part of my journey with this understanding, some remarkable healing has been carried out behind the scenes by healers to close off the provings across time and space.

It also makes me wonder about the length of time we can spend making or proving remedies; I wonder if opening the portals as alchemists for remedy making for only a short time before sealing the portal - just long enough to receive enough information to be able to share the remedy - will maintain an easier process for us all, keeping the energetic fields intact.

I have chosen to work with new remedies in this way, aiming to conduct a trituration and proving in the shortest time possible, and then to energetically close off the proving. I am also reducing how many remedies I am making.

Also, I have started to energetically do the following whenever making or providing remedies. First, I only ever make remedies or conduct provings when connected with the pure unconditional love of Source. I set the intention that this remedy making or proving experience is held safely. I imagine Archangel Metatron taking me to a beautiful space in the cosmos, a completely sealed space - like a cosmic laboratory, in which anything can be done, but the effects are only felt within that container. Mine is a soft light pink room, with soft edges. I have to enter a door that only I can access, and once I am inside, it is sealed. After I have finished, I leave, and ALL the energy of the proving remains inside that space. I go into that space every time I am doing the work on any remedy, After the proving is complete, I ask Archangel Metatron and Source to collapse the space and clear it from existence completely.

The Trituration Journey

Kim Kalina and Canadian Naturopathic Doctor Dr Paul Anderson Theriault have discovered that triturating remedies up to c28 sends the energy of the remedy through different layers of consciousness.

Trituration – the process of making remedies that Dr Hahnemann described – involves mixing, grinding and scraping a substance in a pestle and mortar for an hour at a time for each increase in potency. Trituration usually stops at 2c or 3c before remedies are potentised ("run up") from there.

The Trituration Handbook: into the heart of Homeopathy by Anneke Hogeland and Judy Shriebman[57] describes how triturating up to c4 takes a remedy through all of the layers of a person – physically, emotionally, mentally & spiritually.

57 https://www.homeopathicbooks.com/product/the-trituration-handbook-into-the-heart-of-homeopathy-anneke-hogeland-and-judy-schriebman/

Dr Theriault, in his brilliant book Resurrection of the Vital Force: Blockages to Healing in Homeopathy[58], describes what Kim Kalina discovered in their work in terms of what happens when triturating up to c28 before potentising from there. What they found was that we send the vitality of the remedy beyond the individual (c1-4) into the collective (c5) through family systems miasms, ancestral patterns (c8), countries, civilisations, the planet (c12) the solar system, galaxies, Universe all the way to The Divine (c28).

Epilogue

My sincerest hope and wish is that all of these remedies are able to play their part in bringing healing to our beautiful world.

58 https://www.lulu.com/shop/dr-paul-anderson-theriault-bsc-nd-vnmi/resurrection-of-the-vital-force-blockages-to-healing-in-homeopathy/paperback/product-24368728.html?page=1&pageSize=4

www.ingramcontent.com/pod-product-compliance
Lightning Source LLC
LaVergne TN
LVHW070832220926
848486LV00034B/417/J
* 9 7 8 1 9 1 9 4 5 5 5 0 1 *